Sacroiliac Joint Disorder

Eiichi Murakami

Sacroiliac Joint Disorder

Accurately Diagnosing Low Back Pain

Springer

Eiichi Murakami
JCHO Sendai Hospital
Sendai, Miyagi
Japan

ISBN 978-981-13-1806-1 ISBN 978-981-13-1807-8 (eBook)
https://doi.org/10.1007/978-981-13-1807-8

Library of Congress Control Number: 2018958982

This Springer imprint is published by the registered company Springer Nature Singapore Pte Ltd.
The registered company address is: 152 Beach Road, #21-01/04 Gateway East, Singapore 189721, Singapore

Preface

To be told, "there are no abnormalities detected in your lumbar spine in either an MRI or a CT scan," but to experience pain shortly after sitting on a chair, or to be unable to sleep even on your back, is frustrating. Being unable to perform at work or often being absent from your company can cause your work relationships to suffer. At home, your family, who ought to be your last refuge, often ask, "Are you *really* in pain?" You have been gradually becoming isolated and are finding yourself in a situation where there seems to be no light at the end of the tunnel and are now in a depressed state.

It is estimated that many people who suffer from undiagnosed low back pain can be found all over the country.

Most patients who consult the JCHO Sendai Hospital, to which the author belongs, have experienced a similar path to finding treatment.

When the patient understands that the pain is derived from the sacroiliac joint, based on the effect of the injection, half of the trouble will be solved. It is impressive that some patients say, "It is enough for me to finally know the cause of the low back pain" and they do not wish for any kind of medical treatment.

Their words express that how long and how heavily they have suffered from undiagnosed back pain.

Pain in the sacroiliac joint, with no abnormal findings detected in MRI, CT, etc., accompanies the tragedy in which many patients are not easily diagnosed and may be introduced to psychiatric or psychosomatic medicine.

I first realized 23 years ago that sacroiliac joint pain was undeniably a source of low back pain. Since then, we have treated more than 4000 patients with sacroiliac joint pain.

However, in the beginning, most clinical opinions seemed to agree that the sacroiliac joint is not mobile and thus must not cause pain. Since we announced that there were patients who could return to work after the fusion of the sacroiliac joint, the number of physicians who consider the sacroiliac joint to be a source of the low back pain has been gradually increasing.

The Japanese Sacroiliac Joint Research Society was founded in November 2009, and we have already had seven annual meetings. Physicians including orthopedic surgeons, neurosurgeons, pain clinicians, and medical staff who have an interest in sacroiliac joint pain are increasing in number in Japan.

In order to allow physicians to recognize the existence of sacroiliac joint pain, it is most useful for them to actually experience the effect of the sacroiliac joint injection. For this purpose, my book was published in Japan in 2012 to introduce our method of diagnosis and injection for sacroiliac joint pain.

These days, in the USA and Europe, new methods of sacroiliac joint fusion have been developed, such as the iFuse implant system and DIANA. Furthermore, more than 32,000 patients, mainly in the USA and Europe, have already undergone sacroiliac joint fusion using the iFuse implant system since 2009, which the North American Spine Society (NASS) recommends. Attention paid to sacroiliac joint pain has been increasing in the world.

Based on the idea that anywhere in the world, even at a clinic on an isolated island, the diagnosis and treatment of sacroiliac joint pain (disorder) can be performed, while referring to this book. I set out to write this book.

I pray deeply that this book will be useful for physicians who treat patients suffering from undiagnosed low back pain and a day will come when the correct diagnosis and treatment of sacroiliac joint disorder is carried out all over the world.

Sendai, Japan Eiichi Murakami
2018

Acknowledgements

I would like to express my thanks to Daisuke Kurosawa who is my colleague in Low Back Pain and Sacroiliac Joint Center and helps me with his best and Toshimi Aizawa is an associate professor in the Department of Orthopedic Surgery at Tohoku University School of Medicine, except for whose help, my articles could not be published. Finally, I would like to express my heartfelt gratitude to my mentor in life, SGI President Daisaku Ikeda.

Contents

About the Author

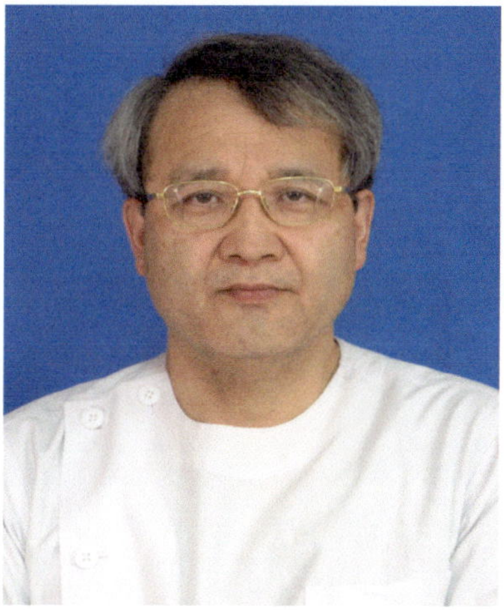

Eiichi Murakami

Brief profile

In 1954, I was born in Iwate, Japan.

In 1981, I graduated from Tohoku University School of Medicine.

In 1982, I started working for the Department of Orthopedic Surgery, Tohoku University School of Medicine.

In 1990, an assistant at the Tohoku University Hospital.

In 1996, vice president of Kamaishi Municipal Hospital.

In 2008, vice president of Sendai-Shakai Hoken Hospital.

In 2014, vice president of JCHO Sendai Hospital.

Since 2009, representative director of the Japanese Sacroiliac Joint Research Society.

Since 2010, chief of Low Back Pain and Sacroiliac Joint Center.

Since 2012, clinical professor of Tohoku University School of Medicine.

My book with the title *Sacroiliac Joint Pain—Undiagnosed Low Back Pain* (in Japanese) was published by the Nankodo Co., Ltd in 2012.

1 The Sacroiliac Joint (SIJ) Has Been Forgotten from History

Abstract

- Non-specific low back pain, not diagnosed by image findings, makes up 85% of low back pain.
- In actuality, gluteal or leg symptoms from ligaments are more common than those from damaged lumbar nerve roots.
- Though the SIJ has been forgotten from history, many people have been suffering from pain of the SIJ.

1.1 Causes of Low Back Pain

1.1.1 Classification

Causes of low back pain are roughly classified into organic factors and nonorganic factors. Organic factors include spondylogenic, neurogenic, viscerogenic (the digestive, urinary, or gynecological system), and vascular factors, while nonorganic factors include psychiatric and psychosocial problems [1].

On the other hand, low back pain is classified into specific low back pain with neurological symptoms and non-specific low back pain without neurological symptoms. Deyo and Weinstein [2] reported that non-specific low back pain, which cannot be given a precise pathoanatomical diagnosis, makes up 85% of patients with isolated low back pain.

Following the progress of imaging equipment such as MRI, etc., we tend to think that the image findings obtained from them directly reveal the cause of low back pain, but that is not always the case. As White and Gordon [3] indicated, the association between symptoms and imaging results is weak. Thus, we should keep in mind that diagnostic imaging is only an auxiliary means to understand symptoms and careful examination of physical findings is necessary in determining whether the findings actually represent the cause of low back pain or not.

E. Murakami, *Sacroiliac Joint Disorder*,
https://doi.org/10.1007/978-981-13-1807-8_1

1.1.2 Pain from Ligaments or Fascias Should Be Much More Common than that from Lumbar Nerve Roots

It is generally thought that leg symptoms develop mainly from damaged lumbar nerve roots. However, as Deyo and Weinstein [2] indicated, lumbar strain or sprain makes up 70% of low back pain, while the prevalence of lumbar disorders with damaged lumbar nerve roots, such as lumbar disc herniation or lumbar canal stenosis, was less than 10% of low back pain. They commented that the most common origins of low back pain are perhaps musculo-ligamentous injuries, degenerative intervertebral discs, and facet joints.

In addition, previously, Hackett [4] indicated that damaged ligaments could produce various leg symptoms (Fig. 1.1). It is important to know that pain from ligaments or fascias is actually much more common than that from damaged lumbar nerve roots. And so, we should pay attention to the possibility that many physicians may misdiagnose referred pain from damaged ligaments as pain from damaged lumbar nerve roots.

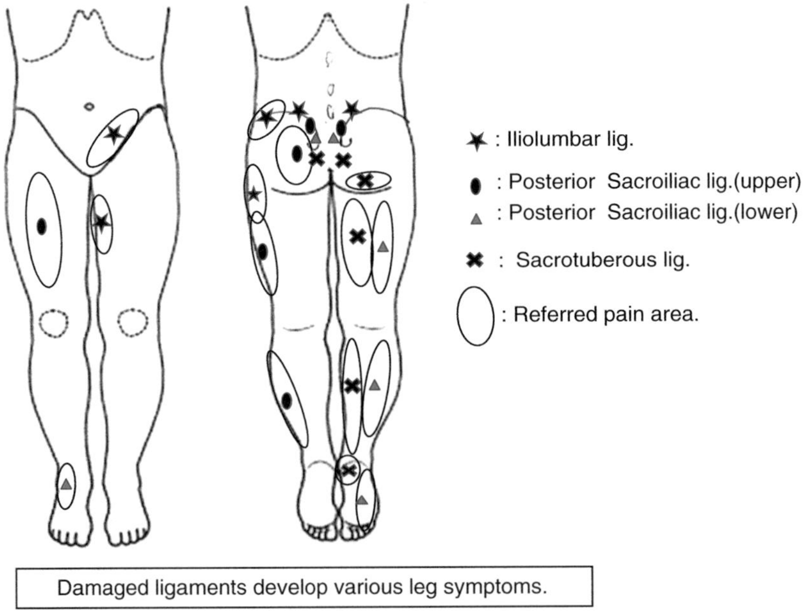

Fig. 1.1 Hackett previously indicated that the iliolumbar ligaments, the posterior sacroiliac ligaments, the sacrosciatic (=sacrotuberous) ligaments should cause referred pain in the thigh, calf, or heel. Modified figure from [4]

Key Message: It Is Natural that Pain from Ligaments or Fascias Is Much More Common

When thinking about the body as if it were a building, it is only natural that the pain from ligaments or fascias is much more common than that from damaged lumbar nerve roots. When earthquakes occur, first the pillars or walls of a building are broken. Then the electric cables and waterworks which are essential to dairy life are usually damaged last by an earthquake. Like a building, the human body is structured so that first, the ligaments or fascias are broken like the walls of a building, when exposed to impacts. And then, the important nerve roots and arteries which are carefully protected by soft tissues are not injured except for severe damage (Fig. 1.2).

Damaged ligaments or fascias cause pain as a warning signal to protect life. If people cannot feel pain like patients with severe diabetes mellitus, their condition will get worse (Fig. 1.3). Pain is very important for protecting life. Considering anatomical structures, it is only natural that pain from ligaments or fascias is much more common than that from damaged nerve roots and arteries.

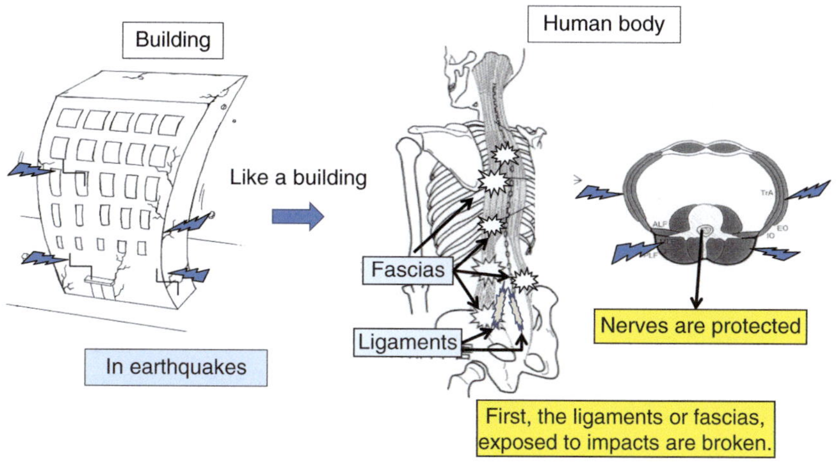

Fig. 1.2 Like a building, the human body is structured so that first, ligaments or fascias, exposed to impacts, are broken, while the essential nerve roots are protected and not injured except by severe impacts

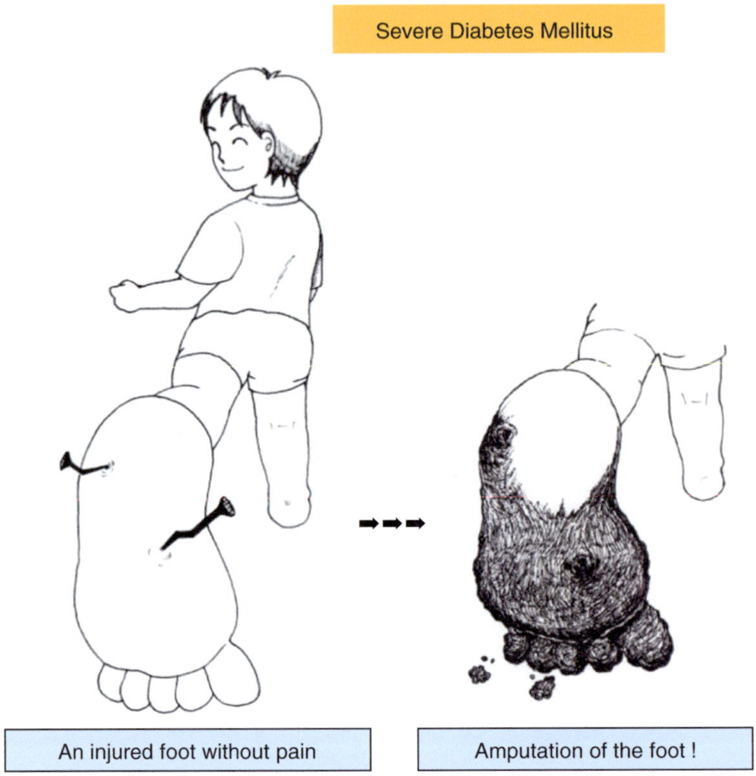

Fig. 1.3 Pain is very important for protecting life. If people cannot feel pain like patients with severe diabetes mellitus, their condition will get worse

1.2 The Forgotten Joint: The Sacroiliac Joint

Interest has been held in the role of the pelvis during childbirth from the times of Hippocrates, but it had long been thought that the sacroiliac joint did not move, under normal condition.

In the early twentieth century in 1905, Goldthwait and Osgood [5] insisted that the sacroiliac joint could cause low back pain and leg pain. As a lot of curettage and drainage of the SIJ was performed at that time for the example of spine caries, it was thought that those symptoms would be associated with the SIJ. However, in 1934, Mixter and Barr [6] reported that lumbar disc herniation pressed on the lumbosacral nerves and induced leg pain. Since then, the most widely accepted cause of lower back and leg pain was shifted to lumbar disc herniation, and the SIJ was forgotten from physicians to manage lower back pain. In the background, it seems that there was some doubt whether the SIJ, capable of hardly any movement, really cause symptoms in the lower limbs. However, regardless of medical disinterest, many people suffering from pain of the SIJ have been existing.

Key Message: Why Did I Started to Study Patients with SIJ Disorder? (Fig. 1.4)
In 1995, I met a woman complaining of severe gluteal and leg pain in Kamaishi City, Iwate Prefecture in Japan. She could not sit on a chair or lay on her back due to pain. She did not respond to any injections including epidural block, selective nerve root block, and facet joint injection. I did not have any idea but injecting into SIJ. I tried SIJ injection, and then her severe pain immediately diminished against my expectation. For the first time, I recognized the existence of SIJ pain. Thus, I estimated that among patients who are diagnosed as having gluteal and leg pain due to lumbar disc herniation, or lumbar spinal stenosis, there should be many whose pain was actually originating from the SIJ. Since then, I have researched the features and treatment of SIJ pain for more than 23 years. I appreciate having met the first woman with SIJ pain.

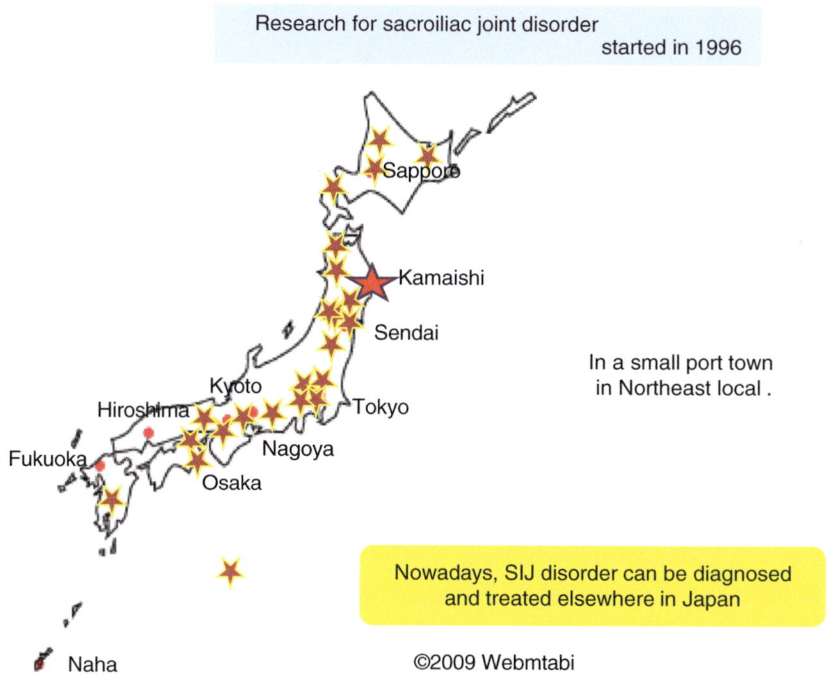

Fig. 1.4 I started studying sacroiliac joint disorder about 23 years ago in a small port town of Kamaishi City in Iwate Prefecture

References

1. Wong DA, Transfeldt E. Macnab's backache. 4th ed. Philadelphia: Lippincott Williams & Wilkins; 2007. p. 19–25.
2. Deyo RA, Weinstein JN. Low back pain. N Engl J Med. 2001;344:363–70.
3. White AA III, Gordon SL. Synopsis: workshop on idiopathic low–back pain. Spine. 1982;7:141–9.
4. Hackett GS. Referred pain from low back ligament disability. AMA Arch Surg. 1956;73:878–83.
5. Goldthwait JE, Osgood RB. A consideration of the pelvic articulations from an anatomical, pathological and clinical standpoint. Boston Med Surg J. 1905;152:593–601.
6. Mixter WJ, Barr JS. Rupture of the intervertebral disc with involvement of the spinal canal. N Engl J Med. 1934;211:210–5.

Basic Understanding of the Sacroiliac Joint

2

Abstract

- The SIJ consists of an articular compartment and a ligamentous compartment.
- Though the range of motion of the SIJ is only a few degrees, the human body would not function well without it.
- The SIJ, which is the only joint parallel to the gravity line, plays a leading role in absorbing vertical loads.
- The SIJ supports upper body weight and absorbs impact from the ground.
- When loaded, the SIJ absorbs load like a damper, while locking instantly and gradually moving.
- Shearing force in the SIJ is prevented by a combination of form closure and force closure.

2.1 Anatomy

2.1.1 Changes of the Pelvis in the Transition from Quadrupedal to Bipedal Walking (Fig. 2.1a, b)

It is well-known that the form of the pelvis has extremely changed, as human evolves from quadrupedal to bipedal walking. In order to enable stable standing and walking, the ilium shortened vertically, and the SIJ moved closer to the hip joint in order to better correspond to the weight load from the upper body and the impact from the floor. In order to stand stably, the spinal column rotated 90° posteriorly, and the SIJ moved just above the hip joint, because rotational moment develops if there is distance between the two joints. In order to support the weight of the upper body, the sacral bones fused and formed the large sacrum, and the

E. Murakami, *Sacroiliac Joint Disorder*,
https://doi.org/10.1007/978-981-13-1807-8_2

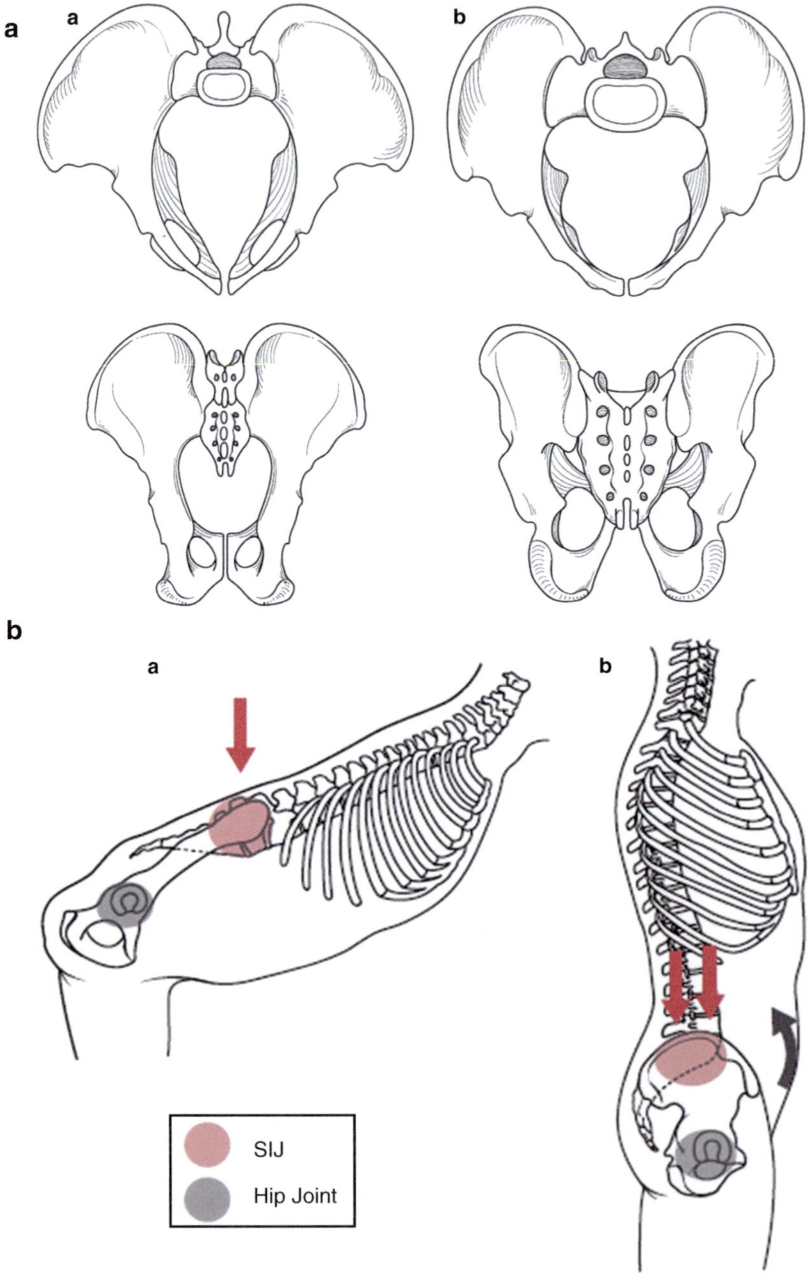

Fig. 2.1 (**a**) *a*: The gorilla. *b*: The human. For the pelvis in humans, compared to that in the gorilla, the sacrum and surface of the SIJ became wider, and the ischium and the pubic bone were shortened. As a result, the SIJ moved closer to the hip joints. With permission from [1]. (**b**) In order to enable bipedal walking, the distance between the SIJ and the hip joint was shortened and the spinal column rotated 90° posteriorly (the black arrow). As a result, the SIJ moved to a location just above the hip joint and changed to be a structure for supporting the weight of the upper body. The red arrow indicates the gravity line. With permission from [1]

Key Message: The Evolution of the Lower Limb: The Lower Limb Is Indicated as the Area from the Ilium to the Foot (Fig. 2.2a)

In the evolution of vertebrates, the pelvic fins of fish transformed into the hind limbs in quadrupedal vertebrates.

The ilium, which did not make contact with the vertebral column in fish or mosasaurs, developed to have a direct connection to the vertebral column in quadrupedal vertebrates such as horses. The hind limbs in quadrupedal vertebrates transformed into the lower limbs in bipedal humans. Therefore, the lower limb is indicated as the area from the ilium to the foot, not from hip joint to the foot.

From this view point, when looking at the SIJ, the importance of the joint in bipedal walking becomes apparent. The sacrum supports the upper body, and the ilium withstands the impact applied to the lower limb from the ground. Thus, it can be easily recognized that the SIJ, connecting the sacrum and the ilium, is always exposed to significant shearing force when walking (Fig. 2.2b).

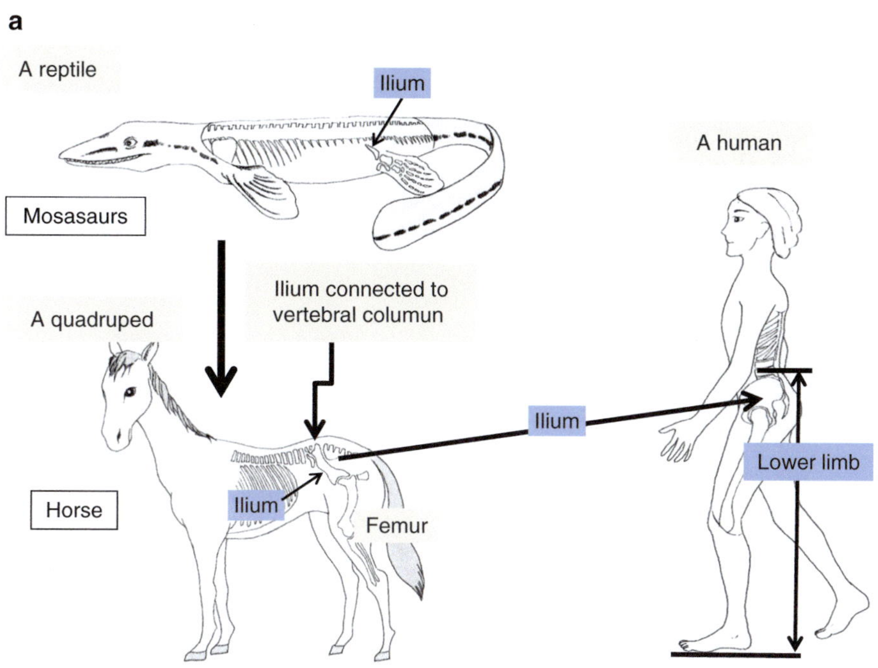

Fig. 2.2 (**a**) The evolution of the lower limb. The ilium connects to the vertebral column in a horse (quadruped). The hind limbs in quadrupedal vertebrates transformed into the lower limbs in humans. The lower limb is indicated as the area from the ilium to the foot. Modified figure from [3]. (**b**) As anatomically most muscles which control lower legs originate from the ilium, the ischium, or the pubic bone. (**a**: posterior view, **b**: anterior view). The SIJ, connecting the sacrum and the ilium, is always exposed to a considerable shearing force when walking

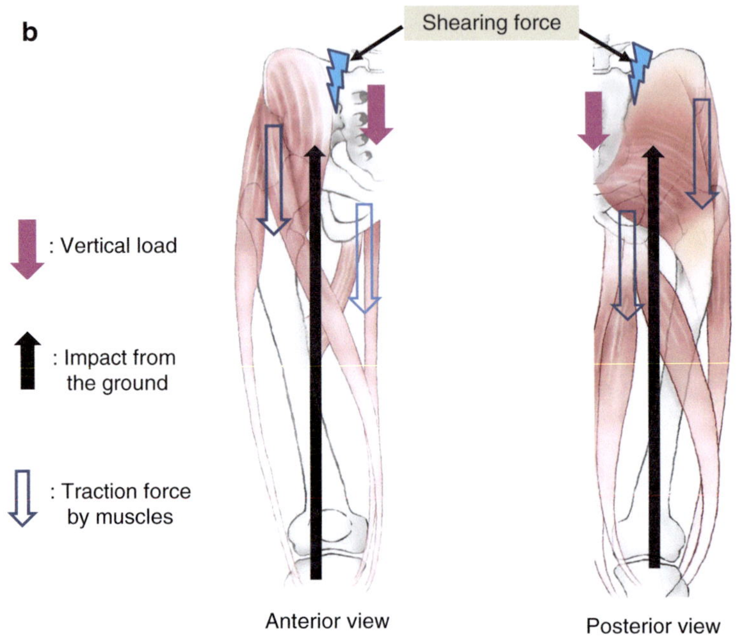

Fig. 2.2 (continued)

ilium expanded horizontally, anteriorly, and posteriorly. The gluteus medius muscle moved to the outside and attached to a proximal portion of the ilium. This prevented the pelvis from tilting while standing on one foot and enabled stable walking. Without these changes, the walking style would have possibly been a Trendelenburg gait [2].

2.1.2 Morphological Anatomy

With gross anatomy, the SIJ forms a joint cavity with the sacrum and the ilium anteriorly. The interosseous sacroiliac ligament and the posterior sacroiliac ligament, which are thought to be the strongest in the human body, occupy the posterior part of the joint (Fig. 2.3). The anterior part of the joint space is covered by the anterior sacroiliac ligament, which is very thin. We found that it was easy to incinerate and remove using bipolar electrocautery in cases of anterior fusion of the SIJ. This finding shows that the anterior pubic syndesmosis is structured to correspond to the load that separates the anterior part of the joint. Based on the

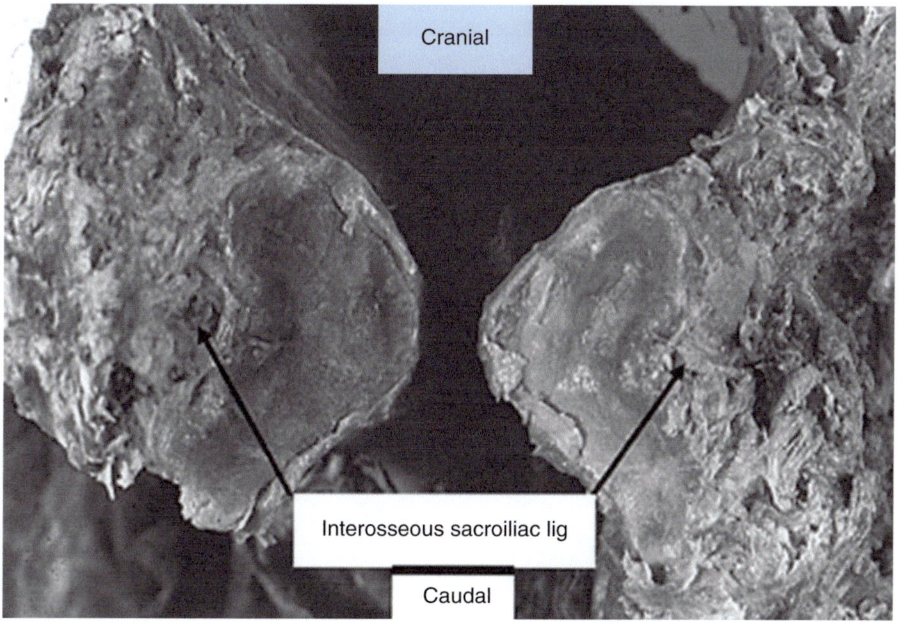

Fig. 2.3 Morphological anatomy of the SIJ. The SIJ forms a joint cavity with the sacrum and the ilium anteriorly. The interosseous sacroiliac ligament and the posterior sacroiliac ligament occupy the posterior part of the joint. With permission from [1]

importance of the ligament group in the back, Bernard et al. defined that the SIJ consists of an articular compartment and a ligamentous compartment [4] (Fig. 2.4). The SIJ has small range of motion, and a load is applied to the two compartments simultaneously.

The joint surface spreads over S1 to S3 and has, anteriorly, a convex auricle, or boomerang shape.

In the neonatal period, the joint surface is narrow and flat, parallel to the sagittal plane, but with a weight load, the sacrum becomes wedge-shaped. In adults, they are V-shaped, opening forward and upward. The joint surface becomes concave on the sacrum side and convex on the ilium side and twists to form an irregular joint cleft [4–6].

As for the joint cartilage, one report says that it is made of "hyaline cartilage" on the ilium side and "fibrocartilage" on the sacrum side [7]. The thickness of the cartilage in adults is 1–3 mm on the sacrum side and less than 1 mm on the ilium side, and so the cartilage of the sacrum side is 2–3 times thicker than that of the ilium side [5, 7, 8].

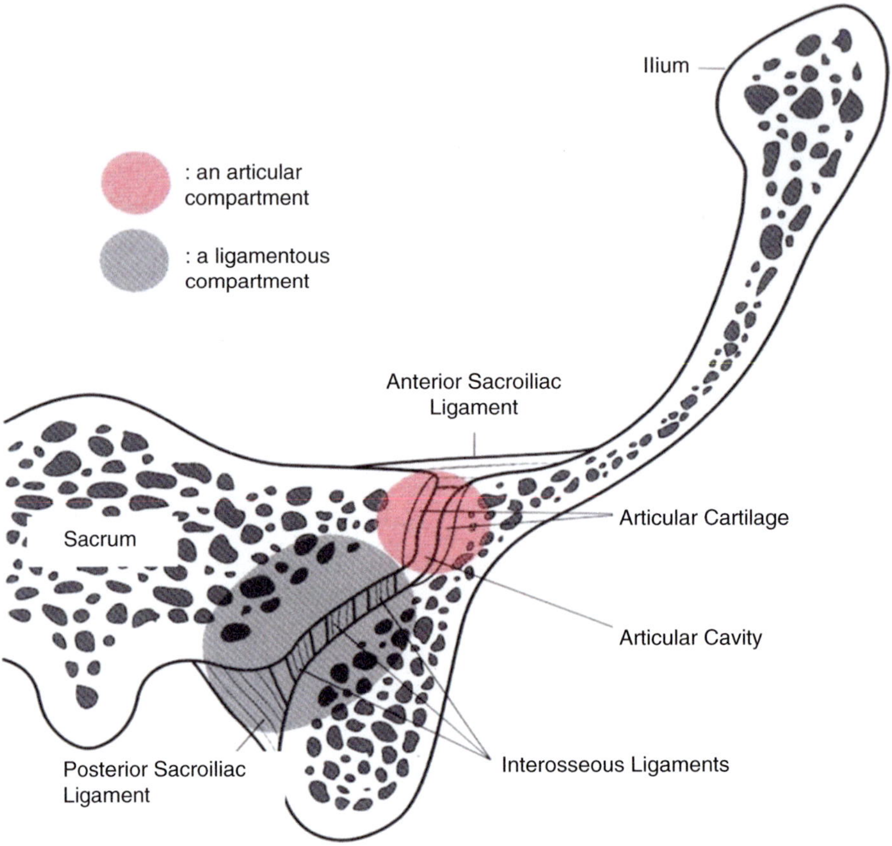

Fig. 2.4 Bernard et al. defined the SIJ as consisting of an articular compartment and a ligamentous compartment

In people over 50 years old, a fusion of the articular surface occurs, but it is partial and fibrous throughout our lives [9]. The anterior part of the joint is covered with a joint capsule, but the rear part of the joint capsule is often undeveloped or insufficient. In that case, the interosseous sacroiliac ligament in the back forms the border of the area [4, 6].

2.2 **Innervation** (Fig. 2.5) [10]

1. The first detailed study of the innervation of the SIJ was done by Solonen [6] in 1957. In the study, all 18 patients had dorsal innervation of the SIJ from the dorsal rami of the S1–S2 nerves. The ventral portion of the joint was

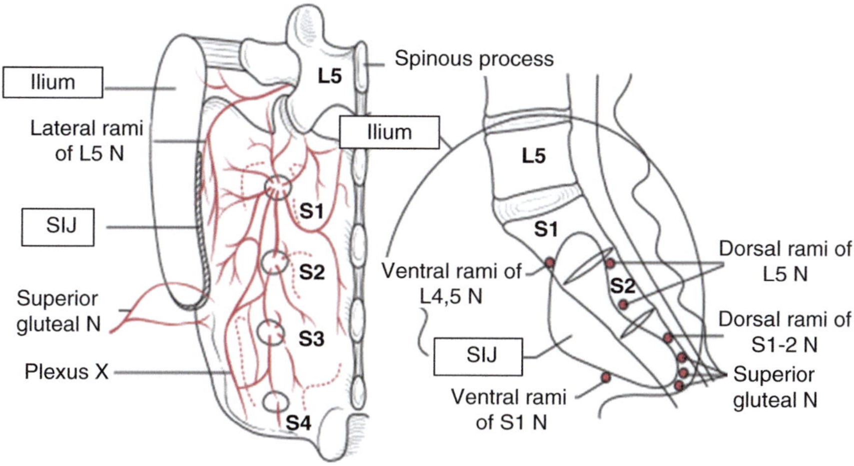

Fig. 2.5 Innervation of the sacroiliac joint

dominantly supplied by the ventral rami of the L4–S2 nerves and the superior gluteal nerve. However, Grob et al. [11] reported that the innervation of the joint was primarily derived from the dorsal rami of S1–S4 nerves and was not confirmed from the ventral ramus of the nerve. Nakagawa's research [12] in Japan suggested that the joint was innervated by the ventral rami of the L4–L5 nerves, from the superior gluteal nerve, and from the dorsal rami of the L5, S1, and S2 nerves. In addition, Ikeda [13] indicated that the superior ventral portion of the joint is innervated mainly by the ventral ramus of the L5 nerve, and the inferior ventral portion of the ventral ramus of the S2 nerve, or branches from the ventral rami of the sacral plexus; the superior dorsal portion is supplied mainly by the dorsal ramus of the L5 nerve, and the inferior dorsal portion is innervated mainly by the dorsal rami of multiple sacral nerves.

2. Broad innervation of the SIJ indicates that pain from the SIJ can develop in any part of the lower back and lower leg. In addition, nerve endings were confirmed in both the capsule of the SIJ [6, 14] and in the dorsal ligamentous area of the joint [12, 14].

In histological studies, Szadek showed the presence of the substance P and CGRP in both the articular cartilage and the posterior ligaments [15, 16]. Sakamoto et al. [17] showed that nociceptors were found in the ligaments and muscles in the dorsal portion of the SIJ in cats and this suggests that the dorsal ligamentous area of the joint can become a source of pain. Both regions can be an origin of SIJ-related pain (Fig. 2.6).

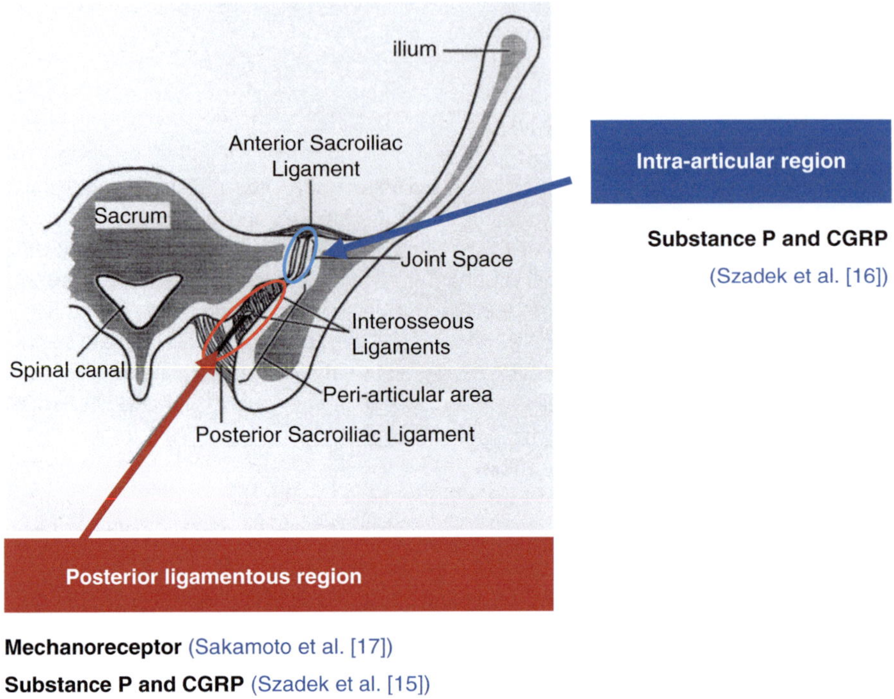

Fig. 2.6 The substance P and CGRP or mechanoreceptor were found in the articular cartilage and the posterior ligaments

2.3 Biomechanics

2.3.1 Structure

The Structure of the SIJ is designed to support very high weight loads. Vertical loads are resisted by (1) the irregular surface of the joint, (2) the wedge-shaped configuration of the sacrum, and (3) the strongest ligaments in the body, such as the posterior sacroiliac ligaments [18]. At any rate, it is true that vertically oriented joints and forward leaning sacrum are not suitable for supporting vertical weight loads. We understand that the posterior ligaments of the joints play an essential role in the support of such loads. The fact that the posterior ligaments are extremely thick shows that the weight load on them is quite large.

2.3.2 Movement

There are still questions regarding the movement of the SIJ. As Kapandji states, classically SIJ has two main motions: so-called nutation where the sacrum bends forward between both ilia around the axis of the posterior ligaments and "counter-nutation"

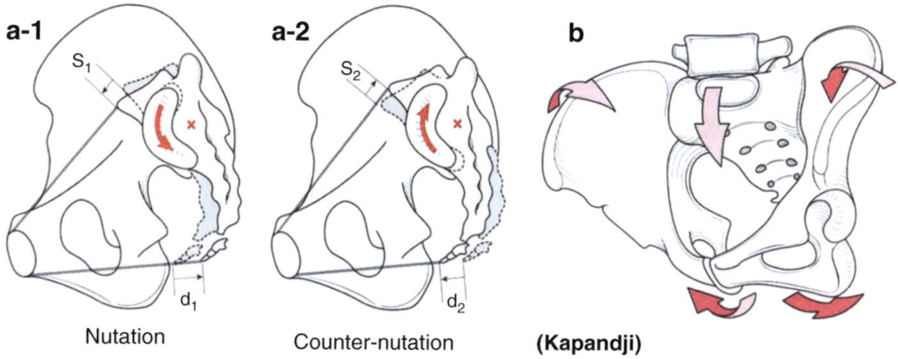

Fig. 2.7 (**a-1**) Nutation, where the sacrum bends forward between both ilia. (**a-2**) Counter-nutation, where the sacrum rises between both ilia. (**b**) Nutation of the sacrum accompanies the closing of both ilia and the separating of both ischial tuberosities. *S1*, *S2*: The distance of movement of the promontorium. *d1*, *d2*: The distance of movement of the coccyx. With permission from [1]

where the sacrum rises posteriorly between the bones (Fig. 2.7a, b) [19], following the movement of the trunk. Although there have been studies done using cadavers, they are less valuable in measuring the motion of the SIJ because cadavers have lost joint reflexes such as the ligamento-muscular reflex [20]. The movement of joints in cadavers is different from that in living bodies. Measurement of the SIJ in the lateral position by Weisl [21] was the first measurement using a living body X-ray. Sturesson et al. [22] utilized the three-dimensional (3D) X-ray measurement method (RSA) developed thereafter. It indicated that in SIJ dysfunction, rotation was very small, 3.9° or less. In addition, translation was only 1.6 mm and rotation was smaller in men than in women, and there were no differences between the symptomatic side and the asymptomatic side. Recent studies are more accurate than RSA.

Nagamoto et al. [23] elucidated the mobility of the SIJ in patients with degenerative lumbar spine disorders compared with healthy volunteers by using in vivo 3D motion analysis with voxel-based registration, more accurate than RSA. As the result, in patients with degenerative lumbar spine disorders, the largest amount of motion occurred around the X axis (accuracy in Rx was 0.00° in previous study), which were the mean rotation angles of 0.57° during trunk flexion and 0.68° during trunk extension. They were significantly greater than 0.07° in flexion and 0.38° in extension for healthy volunteers. We also found movement of 1.5 mm in the cranial-caudal direction (accuracy of 0.1 mm) in the SIJ of patients with SIJ disorder using 3D motion analysis (Fig. 2.8).

2.3.3 Proof of Movement in the SIJ on X-Ray

2.3.3.1 Vacuum Phenomenon

It is quite difficult to show the mobility of the sacroiliac joint in an image. However, it can be understood from vacuum phenomenon occurring in the joint that the

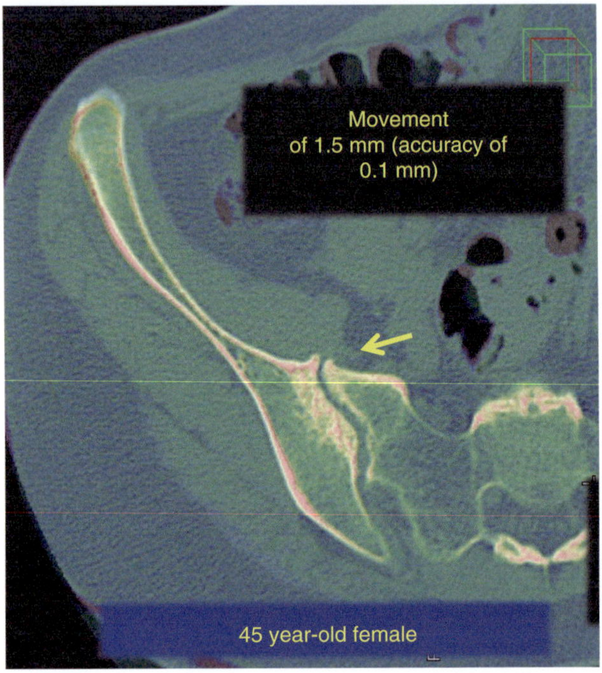

Fig. 2.8 Proof of movement in the cranial-caudal direction in the SIJ using 3D motion analysis. Investigated by Inoue N, Rush University, Medical Center

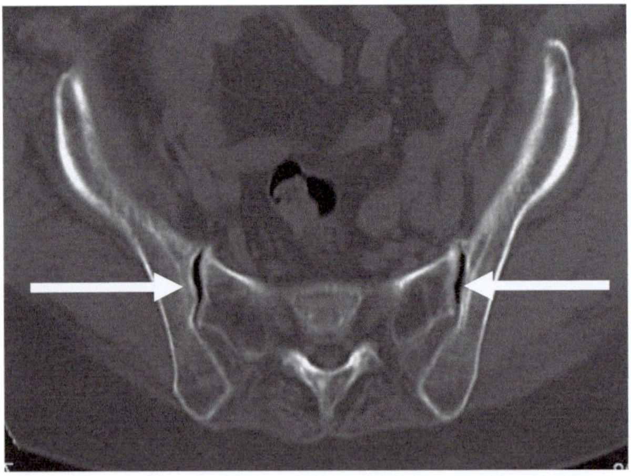

Fig. 2.9 The vacuum phenomenon: the vacuum phenomenon, which is often found, in the SIJ indicates that the joint is a mobile joint. With permission from [1]

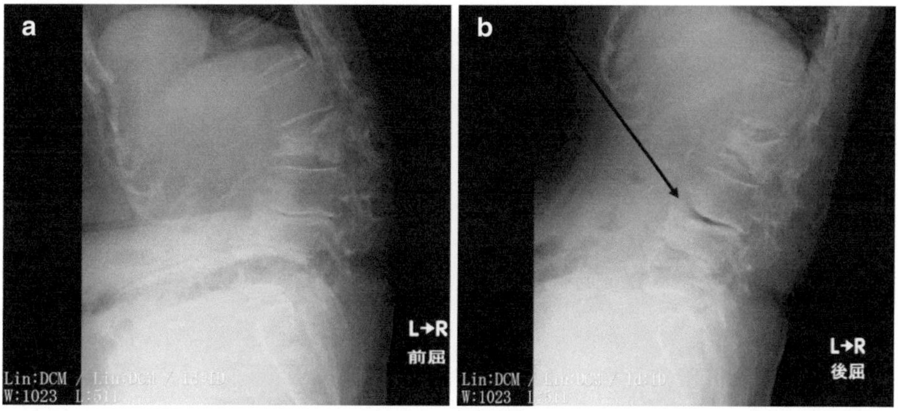

Fig. 2.10 (**a**) Forward bending view of the lumbar spines. (**b**) Backward bending view of the lumbar spines. The vacuum phenomenon in the lumbar intervertebral discs when bending posteriorly shows movement in the lumbar intervertebral spaces. With permission from [1]

sacroiliac joint can move (Fig. 2.9). This phenomenon is by no means uncommon. It is sometimes seen in the lumbar intervertebral disc in X-P and CT images. This phenomenon in the lumbar intervertebral discs is considered to be evidence of the movement in the lumbar intervertebral spaces [24] (Fig. 2.10a, b).

2.3.3.2 Change of Pelvic Incidence

Lee et al. [25] reported that even every one considers that pelvic incidence (PI) is a constant, PI increased in all patients following surgical correction of fixed lumbar lordosis. They revealed that the mean disparity in PI preoperatively and at last follow-up was 11.4° without sacro-pelvic fixation ($n = 18$) and 5.9° with sacro-pelvic fixation ($n = 11$) ($p = 0.002$); their data indicate a proof of mobile of the SIJ.

Key Message: The SIJ Is Extremely Well-Suited to Bipedal Walking

The surface structure of the sacroiliac joint appears disordered at a glance. However, from the point of view of fluid dynamics, stress dispersion (hydraulic mechanism formation), Yoshida [26] showed that the joint structure (type 9) is best adapted to bipedal walking and that a constant flow of synovial fluid develops when subtly different bulges in the articular surface are subjected to gravity (Fig. 2.11a, b).

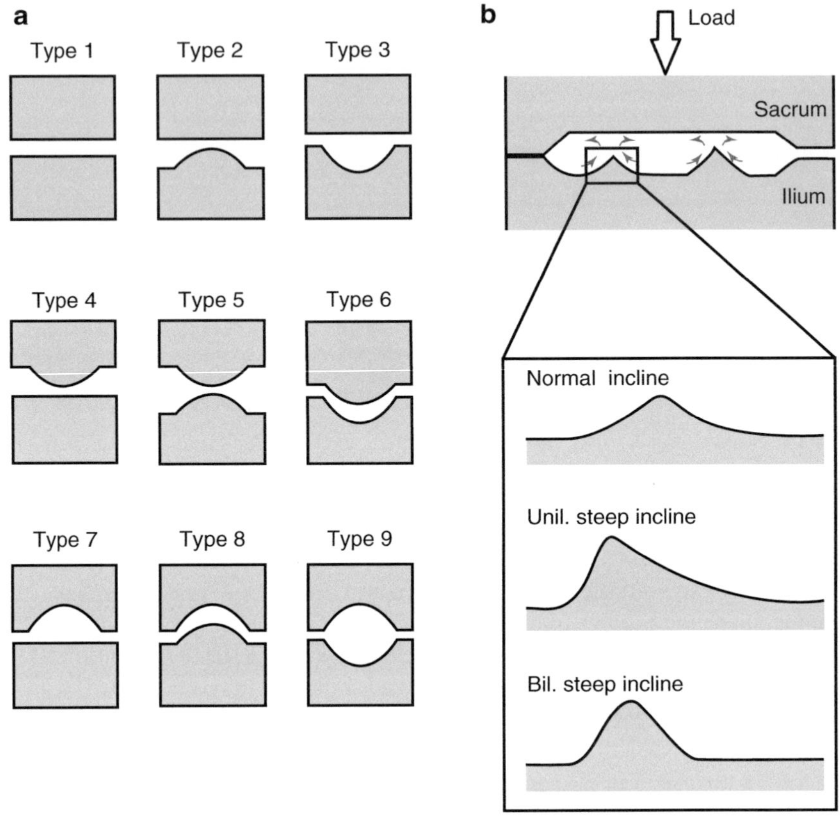

Fig. 2.11 (**a**) Types of joint surfaces. (**b**) Synovial flow when bearing weight. Joint structure type 9 is best adapted to bipedal walking. Subtly different bulges in the articular surface create a constant flow of synovial fluid when bearing a load. With permission from [1]

2.4 Function

2.4.1 Essential Functions to the Human Body

The human body would not function well without the SIJ.

2.4.1.1 Two Types of Synovial Joints

The human body consists of two types of synovial joints which have far different functions. They are classified as gliding joints and amphiarthrosis by their motion pattern [27] (Fig. 2.12).

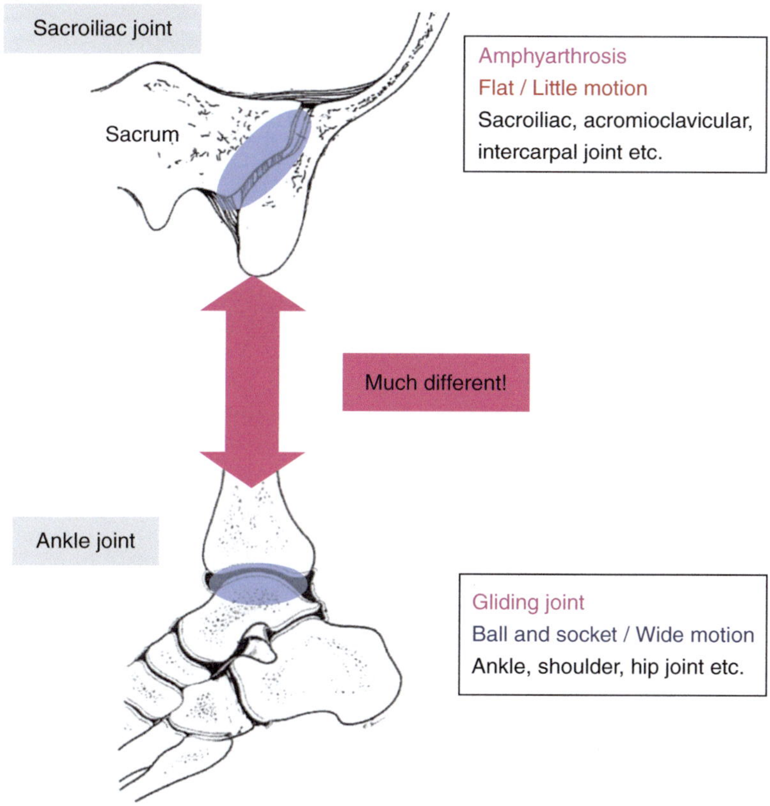

Fig. 2.12 Two types of synovial joints

Gliding joints, including the ankle joint (hinge joint), the shoulder joint (ball joint), and the hip joint (cotyloid joint), have very large ranges of motion. On the other hand, amphiarthroses such as the SIJ, the acromioclavicular joint, and the intercarpal joints are capable of very little movement and are surrounded by thick ligaments. When generally speaking of joints, we may imagine only gliding joints. However, we should keep in mind that it is not only the gliding joints that allow the human body to function well. The amphiarthrosis also plays an important role in absorbing impacts applied to the human body, while moving slightly as the articular surfaces slip.

2.4.1.2 The SIJ, Parallel to the Gravity Line, Plays a Leading Role in Absorbing Vertical Loads

The SIJ is the only joint that runs parallel to the gravity line among the various joints that bear vertical loads.

The human body consists of the intervertebral discs and joints such as the atlantoaxial joint, the SIJ, the hip joint, the knee joint, and the ankle joint to absorb the

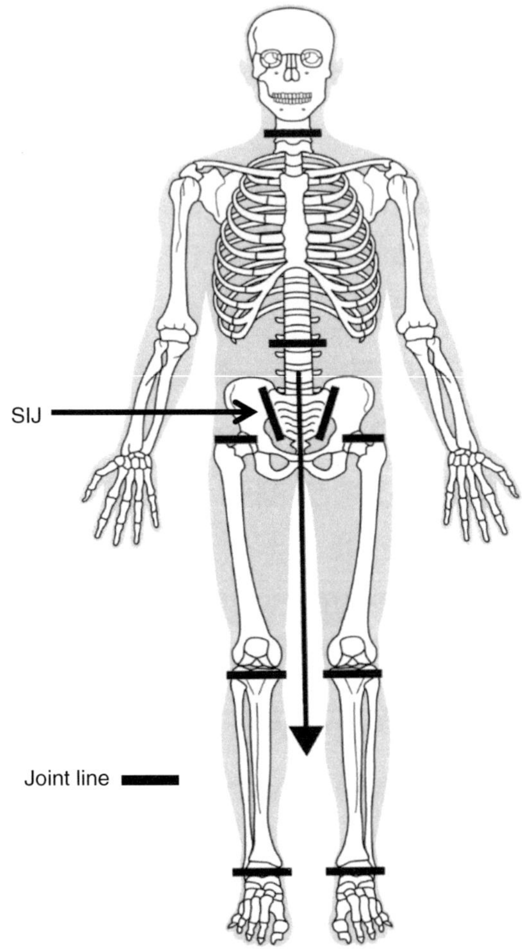

Fig. 2.13 Among the various joints that bear vertical load, only the SIJ runs parallel to the gravity line

impacts applied to it. However, only in the SIJ does the joint line run roughly parallel to the gravity line. The intervertebral discs and the joints that cross at right angles to the load line do not biomechanically play a main role in absorbing vertical impacts. This means that the SIJ, which runs parallel to the gravity line, plays a leading role in absorbing vertical loads (Fig. 2.13).

2.4.1.3 The Main Functions of the SIJ: Supporting the Upper Body and Absorbing the Impact from the Ground

The SIJ supports the upper body, which accounts for about 2/3 of the full weight of the body, and absorbs the impact from the ground with a little joint motion when kicking, jumping, or running. The joint responds to these various actions with only several mms of movement in the joint (Fig. 2.14).

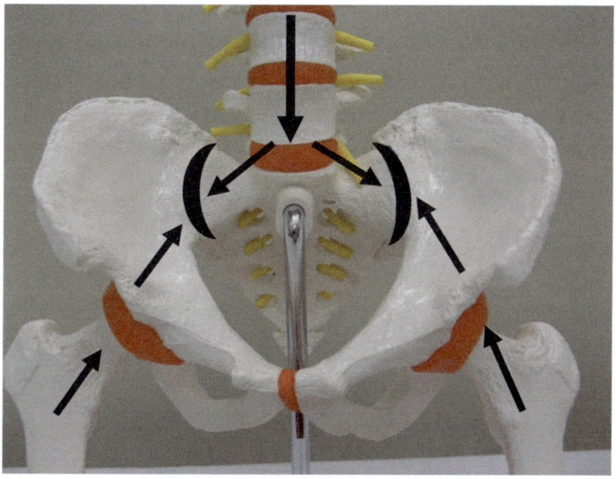

Support and absorb the load

Fig. 2.14 The SIJ supports the upper body as well as absorbs the impact from the ground with little joint motion

2.4.2 Specific Movements of the SIJ for Absorbing Impact

2.4.2.1 Ligamento-Muscular Reflexes

In 1958, Palmar [20] was the first to report on the existence of reflexes between ligaments in a joint and the muscles acting on that joint. The effect of direct tension on the medial collateral ligament of the knee resulted in fast reflex response in periarticular muscles, which is interpreted as joint protective reflexes. Since then, similar studies on joint ligamento-muscular reflexes in humans have been documented in the ankle [28], elbow [29], knee [30], shoulder [31], and recently wrist joint [32] (Fig. 2.15). Evidence of proprioceptive reflexes between wrist ligaments and forearm muscles has recently been presented [32]. After stimulation of the scapholunate interosseous ligament, there is an immediate response in the flexor carpi radialis/ulnaris. Later co-activations of wrist flexors and wrist extensors were observed, likely intended to produce broad wrist stability. For other joints, it is well recognized that a co-contraction of the agonist and antagonist muscles around a joint will create general joint stiffness, thereby effectively reducing the risk of joint damage. It is naturally assumed that similar reflexes exist in the SIJ.

2.4.2.2 Arthrostatic Reflex and Arthrokinetic Reflex

For joint reflexes, Wyke31 has confirmed that there are four types of joint sensory receptors in the joint capsule and ligaments (Table 2.1). Type I and II are important for the movement of the joint. Type I is related to the reflex that causes the joint to become hard when an external force is applied. This is called the

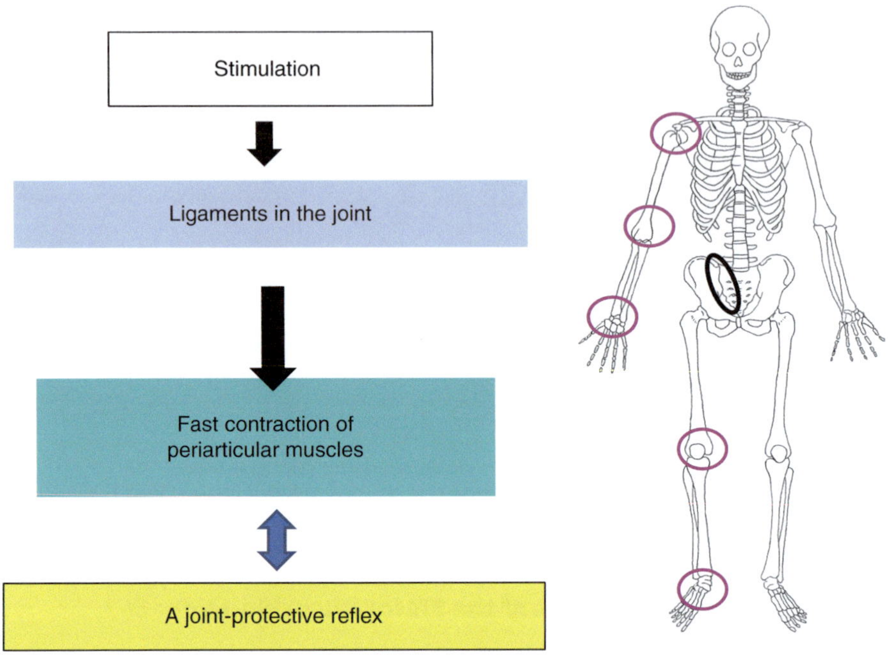

Fig. 2.15 Ligamento-muscular reflexes. Ligamento-muscular reflexes in humans, where stimulation on ligaments of the joint induces fast reflective contraction of periarticular muscles, have already been documented in the shoulder, elbow, wrist, knee, ankle joint. Similar reflexes can exist in the SIJ

Table 2.1 Characteristics of articular receptor systems [33]

Type (receptor)	Location	Behavioral characteristics
I: Ruffini	Fibrous capsules of joints (in superficial layers)	Static and dynamic mechanoreceptors: low-threshold, slowly adapting
II: Paccini	Fibrous capsules of joints (in deeper subsynovial layers), articular fat pads	Dynamic mechanoreceptors: low-threshold, rapidly adapting
III: Golgi	Applied to surfaces of joint ligaments (collateral and intrinsic)	Dynamic mechanoreceptors: high-threshold, slowly adapting
IV: (a) Tridimensional plexuses of unmyelinated nerve fibers (b) Free unmyelinated nerve endings	Fibrous capsules of joints. Articular fat pads Joint ligaments (collateral and intrinsic)	Nociceptive mechanoreceptors: very high-threshold, non-adapting

"arthrostatic reflex." Subsequently, the movement of the SIJ is regulated. This is called the "arthrokinetic reflex." In this subsequent reflex, the Type I and II sensory receptors play the main role (Table 2.2). A shellfish closes instantly when touched; this reaction is similar to the arthrostatic reflex of the SIJ. The SIJ hardens instantly when a load is applied, like a shellfish. For shellfish, it next gradually opens by continuously applying a small amount of force; this reaction is similar to the arthrokinetic reflex (Fig. 2.16). We have the impression that the SIJ does not move, due to the arthrostatic reflex instantly making the joint hard when a load is applied. In this way, the SIJ begins to move like a snail by a small continuous force (Fig. 2.17a). When bending forward, it is supposed that the sacrum gradually begins to bend (nutation), as the lumbar vertebrae bend forward (Fig. 2.17b).

Table 2.2 Joint receptor reflex

1. Arthrostatic reflex—Type I receptors play the main role
Increase: Hypertension in the soft tissues and muscles. Decrease of play in the joint. Repeated hypertension in the joint soft tissues
Decrease: Hypotension in the soft tissues and muscles. Increase of play in the joint
2. Arthrokinetic reflex—Type I and II receptors play the main role. The joint is regulated in its movement
Increase: Spasticity of muscles. Increase of muscle rigidity
Decrease: Loss of muscle contractive power, absence of reflective muscle contraction

Type I receptors are related to the arthrostatic reflex that causes the joint to become hard when an external force is applied. The movement of the SIJ is regulated by the arthrokinetic reflex. Type I and II sensory receptors relate

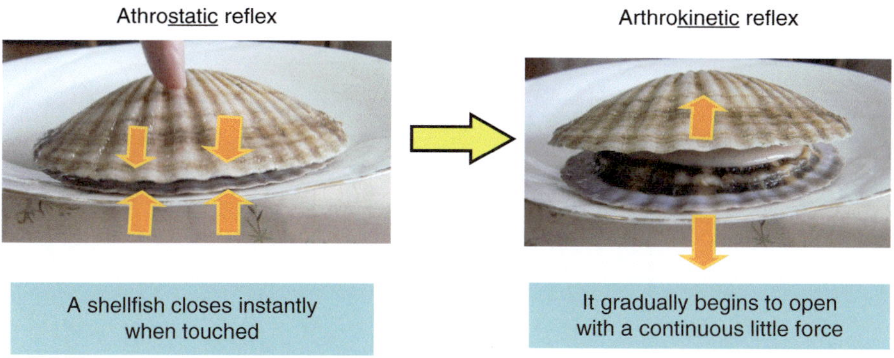

Fig. 2.16 Specific reaction of the SIJ. A shellfish closes instantly when touched; this reaction is called the arthrostatic reflex. The SIJ is also hardened instantly when bearing a load like a shellfish. The shellfish then opens gradually with a slight continual force. This reaction is called the arthrokinetic reflex and the SIJ behaves in the same way

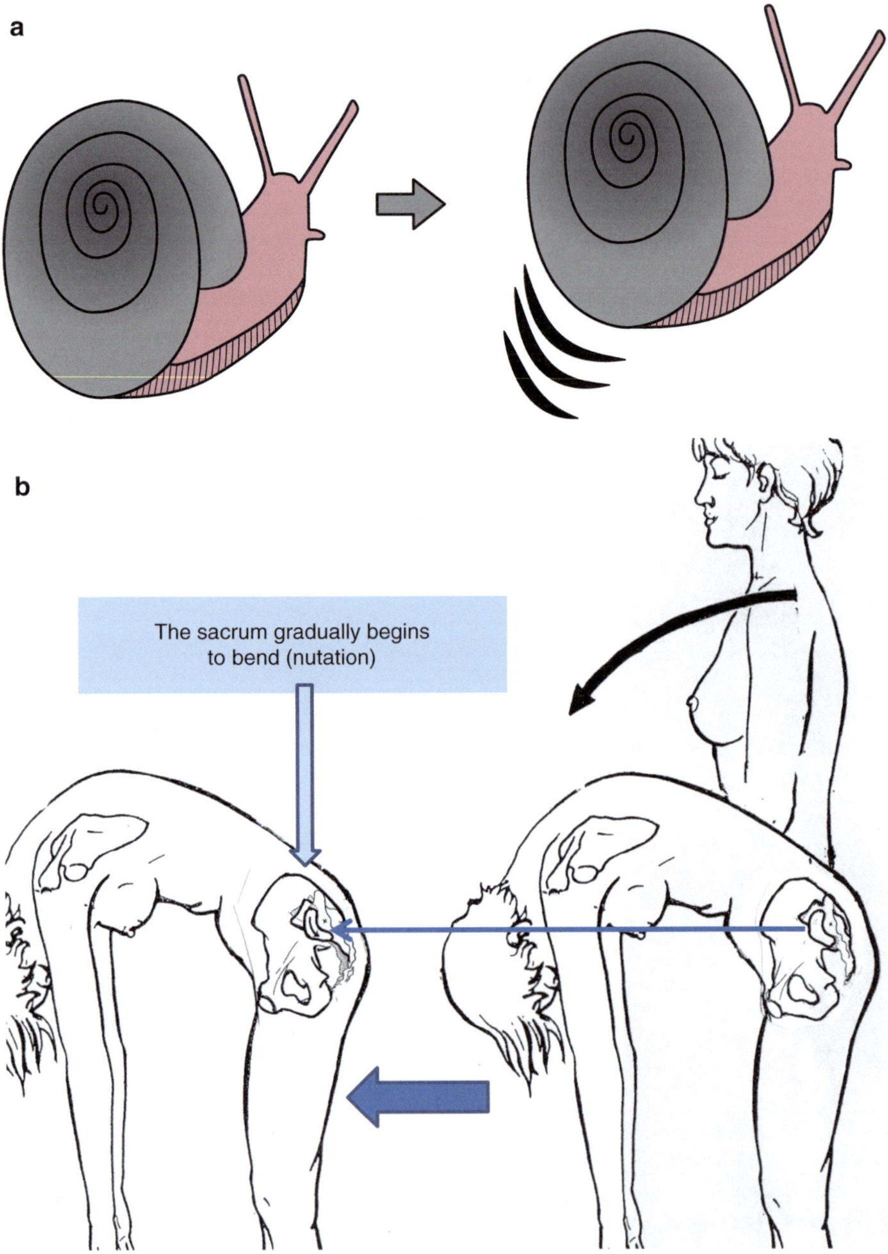

Fig. 2.17 (**a**) In this way, the SIJ starts to move similar to a snail. With permission from [1]. (**b**) The sacrum gradually begins to bend (nutation), as lumbar spines bend forward

In cases of SIJ disorder, forward bending is hindered after a certain degree due to immobility of the SIJ joint.

2.4.2.3 The SIJ Functions Characteristically Like a Damper

When a load is applied, joints such as the SIJ or subtalar joint are locked instantly and then gradually move. This reaction absorbs the load like a damper (Fig. 2.18). If amphiarthrosis acting like dampers did not exist, it would be impossible for children to jump down from trees and immediately begin running without injury (Fig. 2.19). Thus, it can be seen that the human body is kept free from injury thanks to the many amphiarthrosis, such as the SIJ. These joints are distributed throughout the body and absorb impacts exquisitely.

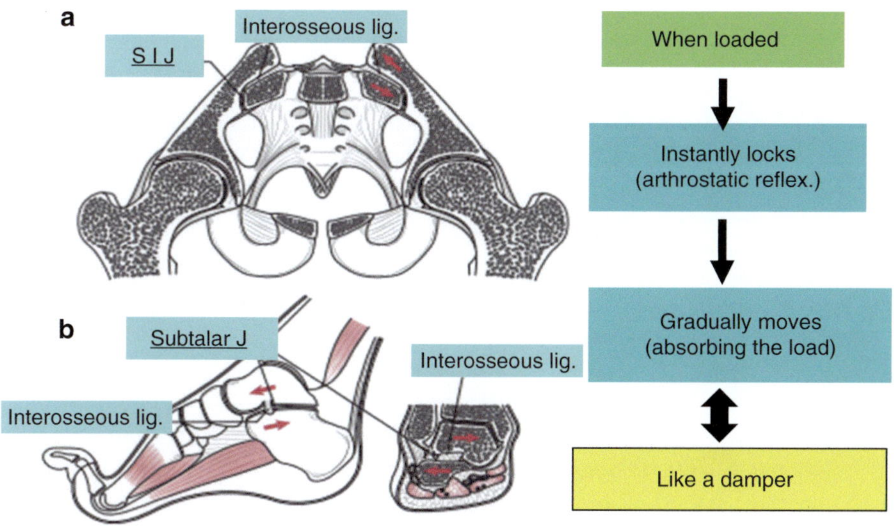

Fig. 2.18 A characteristic function of the SIJ like a damper. It is supposed that joints such as the SIJ (**a**) or subtalar joint (**b**) act like a damper. With permission from [1]

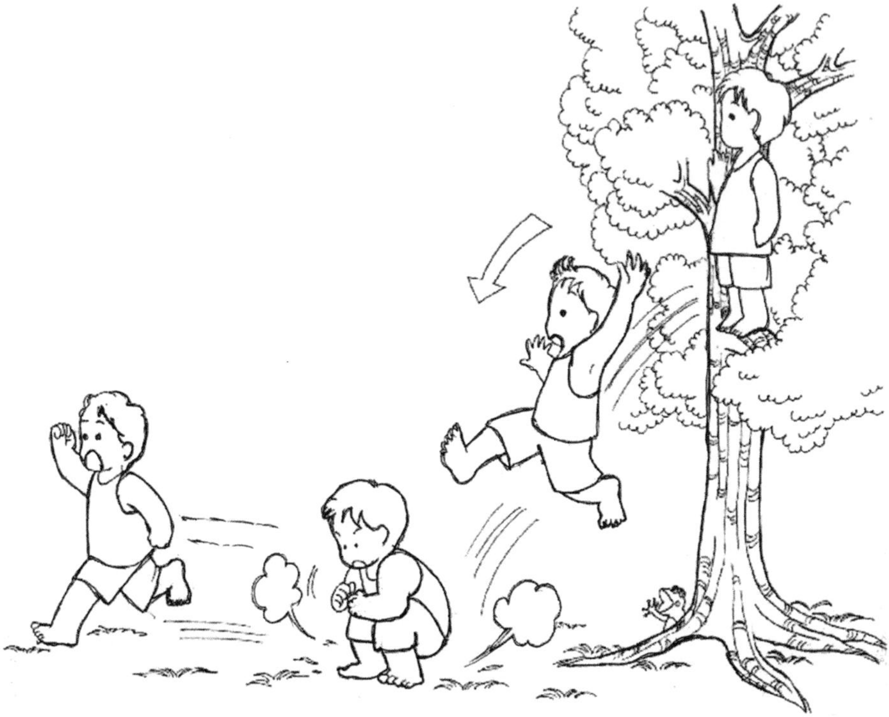

Fig. 2.19 If joints such as the SIJ, acting like dampers, did not exist in the human body, it would be impossible for children to jump down from trees and immediately run without injury

Key Message: Damper: A Shock Absorbing Device (Fig. 2.20a) **and Seismic Isolation Rubber for Shock Absorption** (Fig. 2.20b)

A damper system is utilized in airplanes, automobiles, and buildings. For example, when an airplane lands, the tires would go flat immediately if the impact were received directly through the wheel. But in actuality, the impact is absorbed using a shock-absorbing device called a damper. In a damper, when force is applied to the piston rod, high viscosity oil passes through an orifice in the piston. This creates a resisting force and the impact is decreased.

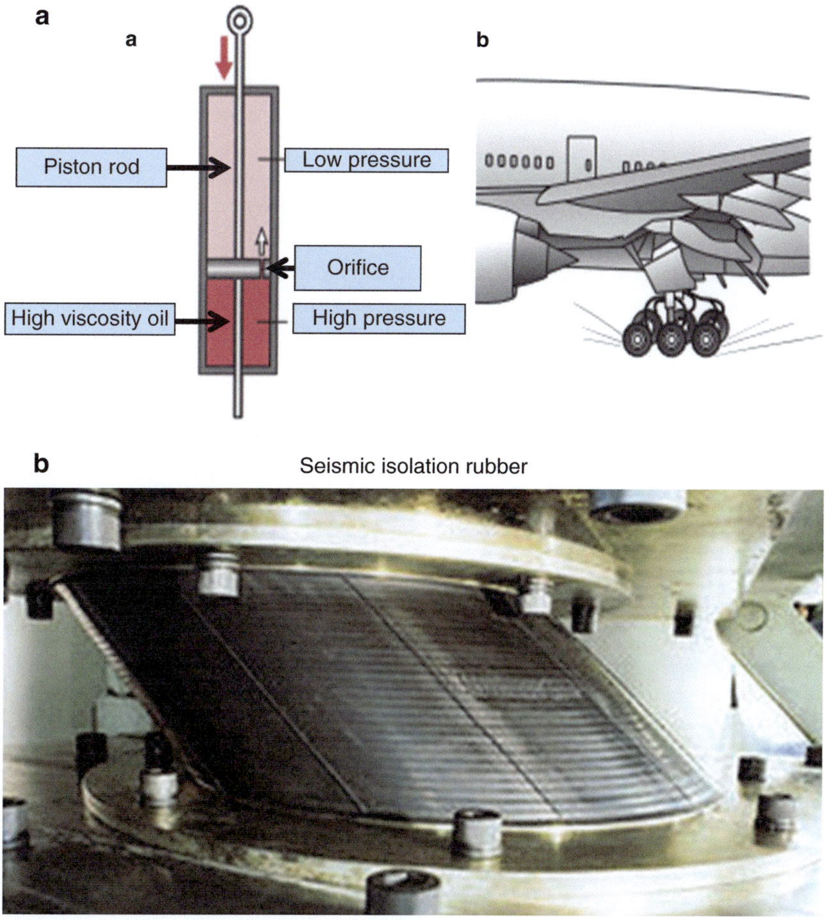

Fig. 2.20 (**a**) Damper: a shock-absorbing device. With permission from [1]. *a*. An impact force which is applied to the piston rod is absorbed by creating a resisting force, while high viscosity oil passes through an orifice in the piston. *b*. A damper is used as a shock-absorbing device to decrease the impact created when an airplane lands. (**b**) Seismic isolation rubber. https://www.bridgestone.co.jp/saiyou/recruit/technology/antiseismic-rubber/index.html

2.4.2.4 The SIJ Easily Causes Joint Dysfunction (Fig. 2.21)

It is inevitable that the SIJ easily causes minor subluxation which leads to dysfunction of the joint when unexpected movement and heavy loads are applied to the joint. This is because the joint has little mobility and so does not have much play.

2.4.3 A Mechanism for Providing the Stability of the Pelvis

2.4.3.1 Form Closure and Force Closure (Fig. 2.22)

Shearing force in the SIJ is prevented by a combination of specific anatomic features (form closure) and compression generated by muscles and ligaments that

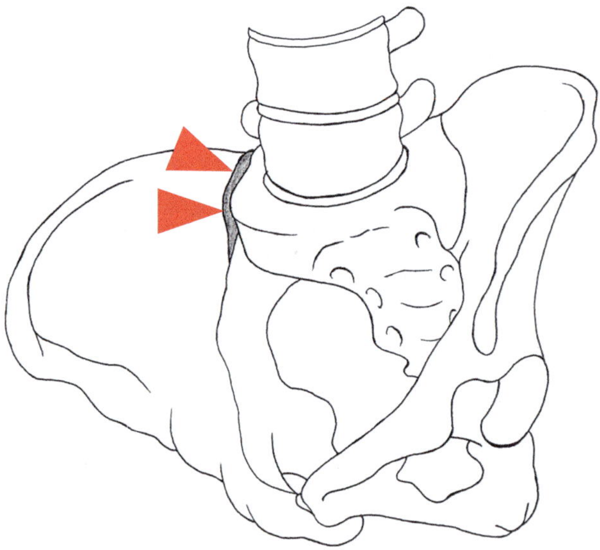

Fig. 2.21 The SIJ, which easily causes joint dysfunction. The SIJ, which bears a big load with little motion, is likely to cause dysfunction, especially when unexpected movement and big load are applied

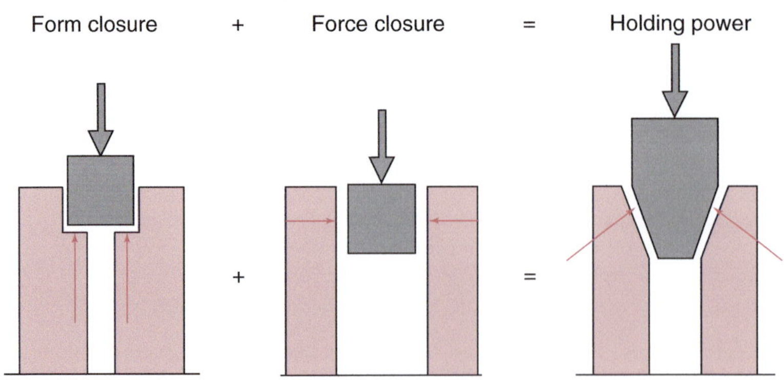

Fig. 2.22 The stability of the pelvis (modified from [34]). The stability of the pelvis is created by a combination of specific anatomic features (form closure) and compression generated by muscles and ligaments (force closure). With permission from [1]

accommodate specific loading situations (force closure) [35]. Form closure depends on the shape of joints, the coefficient of friction, and articular cartilage. Force closure is a compressive force produced by the contraction of muscles around the pelvis in order to hold the position of the sacrum against the force of gravity [34].

2.4.3.2 The Transversus Abdominis Muscle and the Gluteus Maximus Muscle Are Important in Stabilizing the SIJ

Contraction of the transversus abdominis muscles, which attach to the ilium, stabilizes the SIJ, and early activation of the muscles before movement during a variety of functional tasks plays an important role in stabilizing the spine [36]. The gluteus maximum muscles lay across and support the SIJ [37]. Contracting the gluteus maximus muscle can make the sacrotuberous ligament tense and contributes to the stabilization of the SIJ, since the sacrotuberous ligament adheres to the lower part of the gluteus maximus muscle [38].

2.4.3.3 The Inner Unit and the Outer Unit

The two muscle groups are thought to be important for the stability of the SIJs: Two muscle groups play an important role in force closure.

The inner unit consists of the multifidus, the transversus abdominis muscle, the diaphragm, and the pelvic floor. In particular, contraction of the transversus abdominis muscle increases tension in the sacroiliac ligament through the thoracolumbar fascia and strengthens force closure in the SIJ (Fig. 2.23a).

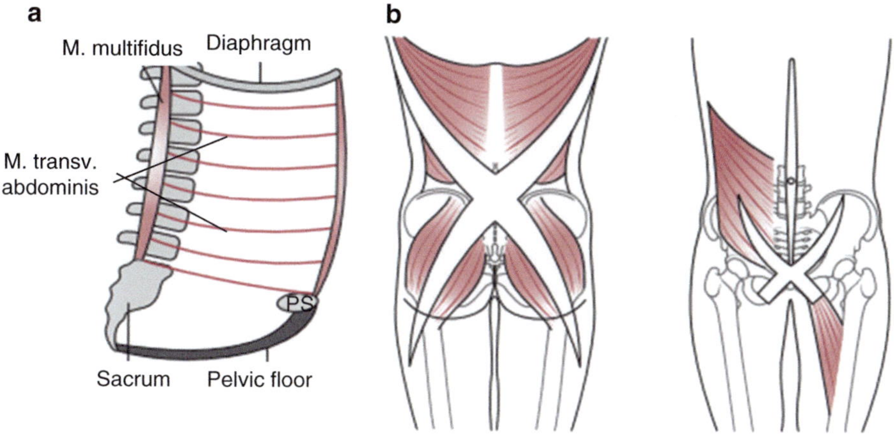

Fig. 2.23 (**a**) The inner unit. The inner unit consists of the multifidus, the transversus abdominis muscle, the diaphragm, and the pelvic floor. Classification of the synovial joints. (**b**) The outer unit. The outer unit consists of four muscle-group systems. The diagram indicates two representative systems, a system which runs obliquely dorsally (the latissimus dorsi muscle and the gluteus maximus muscle) and a system which runs obliquely ventrally (the internal and external oblique abdominal muscle, the thigh adductor muscle on the contralateral side, and the anterior abdominal fascia that connects the muscles). *PS* pubic syndesmosis (modified from [2]). With permission from [1]

The outer unit consists of four systems. One runs obliquely on the dorsal side (the latissimus dorsi muscles and the gluteus maximus muscles). Another system runs obliquely on the ventral side (the internal and external oblique abdominal muscles, the thigh adductor muscle on the contralateral side, and the anterior abdominal fascia that connects the muscles). The third system runs deep vertically along the dorsal side (the spinal erect muscles, the deep chest-spine membrane, the sacrotuberous ligament, and the biceps femoris muscle), and the final system is the lateral system (the gluteus medius/minimi muscle and the thigh adductor muscle on the contralateral side) (Fig. 2.23b).

Key Message: The Long Posterior Sacroiliac Ligament and Sacrotuberous Ligament, Which Control Motion of the SIJ [34]
Sacral nutation is resisted by the sacrotuberous ligament. Counter-nutation of the sacrum tightens the long posterior sacroiliac ligament (Fig. 2.24).

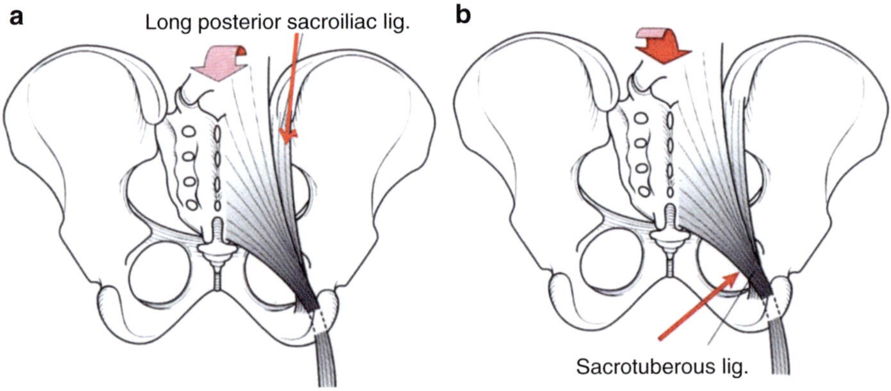

Fig. 2.24 (**a**) counter-nutation of the sacrum is resisted by the long posterior sacroiliac lig. (**b**) nutation of the sacrum is resisted by the sacro-tuberous lig (modified from [34])

References

1. Murakami E. Sacroiliac Joint Pain : Undiagnosed Low Back Pain (in Japanese). Tokyo: Nankodo; 2012.
2. Lee D. The pelvic girdle. 4th ed. London: Churchill Livingstone; 2011. p. 6–8.
3. Radinsky LB. The evolution of vertebrate design. London: The University of Chicago Press; 1987.
4. Bernard TN Jr, Cassidy JD. The sacroiliac joint syndrome: pathophysiology, diagnosis, and management. In: Frymoyer JW, editor. The adult spine: principles and practice. New York: Raven Press; 1991. p. 2107–30.
5. Sashin D. A critical analysis of the anatomy and the pathological changes of the sacroiliac joints. J Bone Joint Surg. 1930;12:891–910.
6. Solonen KA. The sacroiliac joint in the light of anatomical, roentgenological and clinical studies. Acta Orthop Scand. 1957;27(Suppl):1–127.
7. Shunke GB. Anatomy and development of the sacroiliac joint in man. Anat Rec. 1938;72:313–31.
8. Bowen V, Cassidy JD. Macroscopic and microscopic anatomy of the sacroiliac joint from embryonic life until the eighth decade. Spine. 1981;6:620–8.
9. Resnick D, Niwayama G, Georgen TG. Degenerative disease of the sacroiliac joint. Invest Radiol. 1975;10:608–21.
10. Ooseto K, Wakasugi B. Sacroiliac joint block, hip joint block. Surg Ther. 1998;59:341–4. (in Japanese).
11. Grob KR, Neuhuber WL, Kissling RO. Innervation of the sacroiliac joint of the human. Z Rheumatol. 1995;54:117–22.
12. Nakagawa T. A study on the distribution of nerve filaments over the iliosacral joint and its adjacent region in the Japanese. J Jpn Orthop Assoc. 1966;40:419–30. (in Japanese).
13. Ikeda R. Innervation of the sacroiliac joint: macroscopical and histological studies. Nippon Ika Daigaku Zasshi. 1991;58:587–96.
14. Bradley KC. The anatomy of backache. Aust N Z J Surg. 1974;44:227–32.
15. Szadek KM, Hoogland PV, Zuurmond WW, De Lange JJ, Perez RS. Nociceptive nerve fibers in the sacroiliac joint in humans. Reg Anesth Pain Med. 2008;33:36–43.
16. Szadek KM, Hoogland PV, Zuurmond WW, De Lange JJ, Perez RS. Possible nociceptive structures in the sacroiliac joint cartilage: an immunohistochemical study. Clin Anat. 2010;23:192–8.
17. Sakamoto N, Yamashita T, Takebayashi T, et al. An electrophysiologic study of mechanoreceptors in the sacroiliac joint and adjacent tissues. Spine. 2001;26:468–71.
18. White IIIAA, Panjabi MM. The problem of clinical instability in the human spine: a systematic approach. In: Clinical biomechanics of the spine. 2nd ed. Philadelphia: JB Lippincott; 1990.
19. Kapandji IA. The physiology of the joints. In: The trunk and the vertebral column, vol. 3. Edinburgh: Churchill Livingstone; 1974.
20. Palmar I. Pathophysiology of the medial ligament of the knee joint. Acta Chir Scand. 1958;115:312–8.
21. Weisl H. The movements of the sacro-iliac joint. Acta Anat. 1955;23:80–91.
22. Sturesson B, Selvic G, Uden A. Movements of the sacroiliac joints: a roentgen stereophotogrammetric analysis. Spine. 1989;14:162–5.
23. Nagamoto Y, Iwasaki M, Sakaura H, et al. Sacroiliac joint motion in patients with degenerative lumbar spine disorders. J Neurosurg Spine. 2015;23:209–16.
24. Goobar JE, Pote D, Resnick D. Radiography of the hyperextended lumbar spine: an effective technique for the demonstration of discal vacuum phenomena. Can Assoc Radiol J. 1987;38:271–4.
25. Lee JH, Na KH, Kim JH, Jeong HY, Chang DG. Is pelvic incidence is a constant, as everyone knows? Changes of pelvic incidence in surgically corrected adult sagittal deformity. Eur Spine J. 2016;25:3707–14.
26. Yoshida K. Structural medical science: Shizenchiyu no kagi wa juryoku ni aru! Tokyo: Enterprize; 1999. p. 29–109. (in Japanese).

27. Williams PL. Gray's anatomy. 38th ed. New York: Churchill Livingstone; 1995.
28. Freeman MAR, Wyke B. Articular reflexes at the ankle joint: an electro-myographic study of normal and abnormal influences of ankle-joint mechanoreceptors upon reflex activity in the leg muscles. Br J Surg. 1967;54:990–1001.
29. Phillips D, Petrie S, Solomonow M, et al. Ligamentomuscular protective reflex in the elbow. J Hand Surg. 1997;22A:473–8.
30. Tsuda E, Okamura Y, Otsuka H, Komatsu T, Tokuya S. Direct evidence of the anterior cruciate ligament-hamstring reflex arc in humans. Am J Sports Med. 2001;29:83–7.
31. Diederichsen LP, Nørregaard J, Krogsgaard M, et al. Reflexes in the shoulder muscles elicited from the human coracoacromial ligament. J Orthop Res. 2004;22:976–83.
32. Hagert E, Persson JKE, Werner M, L jung BO. Evidence of wrist proprioceptive reflexes elicited after stimulation of the scapholunate interosseous ligament. J Hand Surg Am. 2009;34:642–51.
33. Wyke BD. The neurology of joints: a review of general principles. Clin Rheum Dis. 1981;7:223–39.
34. Vleeming A, Stoeckart R. The role of the pelvic girdle in coupling the spine and the legs: a clinical-anatomical perspective on pelvic stability. In: Vleeming A, Mooney VCJ, Stoeckart R, editors. Movement, stability and lumbopelvic pain. 2nd ed. Edinburgh: Churchill Livingstone; 2007. p. 118.
35. Snijders CJ, Vleeming A, Stoeckart R. Transfer of lumbosacral load to iliac bones and legs. Biomechanics of self-bracing of the sacroiliac joints and its significance for treatment and exercise. Clin Biomech. 1993;8:285–94.
36. Richardson CA, et al. The relation between the transversus abdominis muscles, sacroiliac joint mechanics, and low back pain. Spine. 2002;27:399–405.
37. Hungerford B, et al. Evidence of altered lumbopelvic muscle recruitment in the presence of sacroiliac joint pain. Spine. 2003;28:1593–600.
38. Hungerford B, et al. Altered patterns of pelvic bone motion determined in subjects with posterior pelvic pain using skin markers. Clin Biomech. 2004;19:456–64.

3 Pathophysiology of Sacroiliac Joint Disorder

Abstract

- Repeated heavy exertion, careless lifting of a load, etc. can lead to joint dysfunction.
- SIJ disorder is a common disease which occurs in people of all ages and in both sexes.
- SIJ disorder is classified into two categories which are inflammation in the cavity and joint dysfunction.
- The main origin of SIJ disorder is estimated to be located in the posterior ligamentous area of SIJ.
- Patients with SIJ disorder usually have pain at or around the PSIS, groin, thigh, and leg symptoms not associated with the dermatome of lumbar nerve roots.
- SIJ disorder easily induces pain when sitting, lying in a supine position or on their side (especially on the affected side).
- The imaging methods indicate no findings useful for diagnosing SIJ disorder. Recently, SPECT/CT and ultrasound imaging show abnormal findings in chronic SIJ disorder.

3.1 Pathophysiology and Etiology

3.1.1 Pathophysiology

The SIJ is roughly parallel to the gravity line, so slipping force may occur when vertical load is applied to the joint. The SIJ is in its least packed position (LPP) when bent forward. This posture is supposed to be the most relaxed. Furthermore, the backward bending position of the lumbar spine is called the closed packed position (CPP). In this position the joint is stable and does not easily move [1] (Fig. 3.1).

E. Murakami, *Sacroiliac Joint Disorder*,
https://doi.org/10.1007/978-981-13-1807-8_3

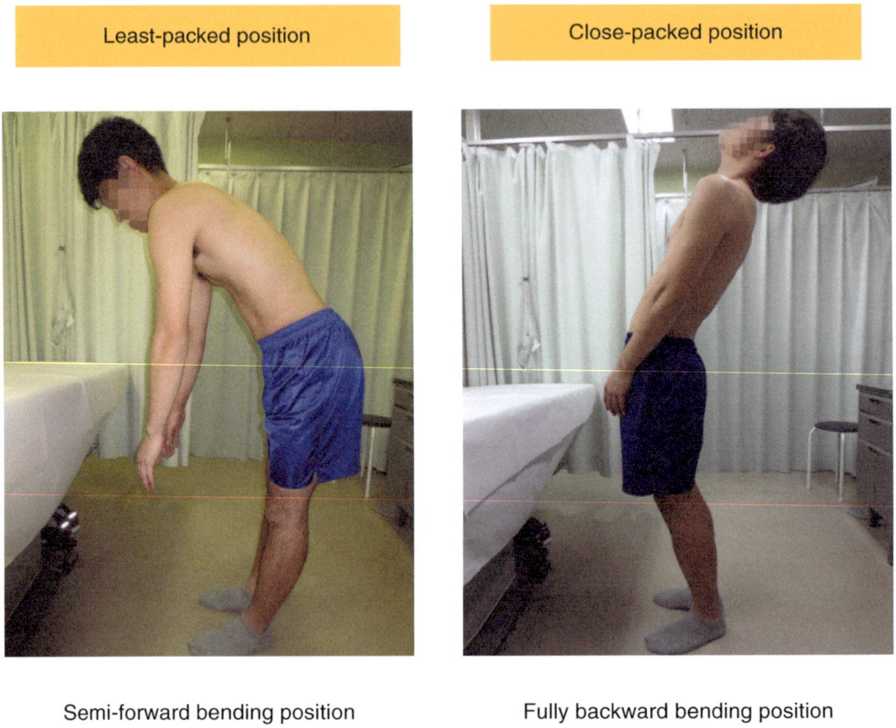

Fig. 3.1 LPP and CPP in the SIJ. Joints generally have a least packed position (LPP), where the joint is most relaxed, and a closed packed position (CPP), where the joint is stable. For the SIJ, the LPP is the forward bending position, and the CPP is the backward bending position of the lumbar spine

Repeated heavy exertion, careless lifting of a load, or twisting of the lumbar spine can cause a failure in the cooperation between the muscles around the pelvis and may cause minor subluxation of the joint, which can lead to joint dysfunction.

Borowsky et al. [2] indicated that both peri-articular and intra-articular injections were effective for patients with SIJ disorder rather than only an intra-articular injection. Therefore, it is should be true that there is a pain origin of SIJ disorder in not only the peri-articular area but also the intra-articular area. If patients are diagnosed using only intra-articular injections, there is a strong possibility that the total number of patients with SIJ disorder would be underestimated. In our study [3] a peri-articular injection was more effective than an intra-articular injection for patients with SIJ disorder. Thus (so), it can be assumed that the main origin of SIJ disorder is located in the posterior ligamentous area of the SIJ.

We imagine the mechanism of pain appearance from joint dysfunction as follows: When minor subluxation accidentally occurs in the joint, the hypertension of the posterior ligament can originate. Then the nerve endings in the ligament can respond and induce SIJ pain (Fig. 3.2).

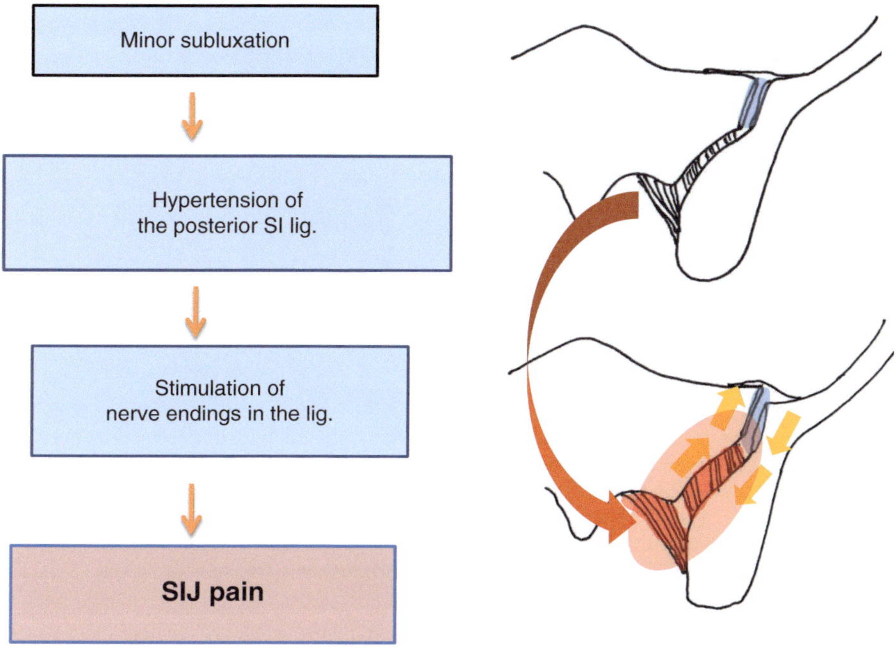

Fig. 3.2 The pain mechanism originating from joint dysfunction. Minor subluxation occurring in the SIJ creates hypertension of the posterior ligament. This can cause the nerve endings in the ligament to be stimulated and induce pain

Key Message: Causes for Increasing SIJ Disorder: Lack of Walking or Chair Life in Modern Times [1]

1. Lack of walking

   If the patient is walking enough every day and physiologically upright bipedal walking is achieved, strains are absorbed, and distortion is also automatically restored even if the cervical spine and pelvis deviate somewhat from the gravity line. However, when walking exercise is insufficient, distortion of the body is not restored, and it falls to a morbid condition [4].
2. Chair life

In the pelvis, when you stand, a closing force is at work, and when you sit on a chair without lumbar support, the weight of the trunk allows the sacrum bend forward (nutation). Then, the pelvis opens easily and becomes unstable [4, 5] (Fig. 3.3).

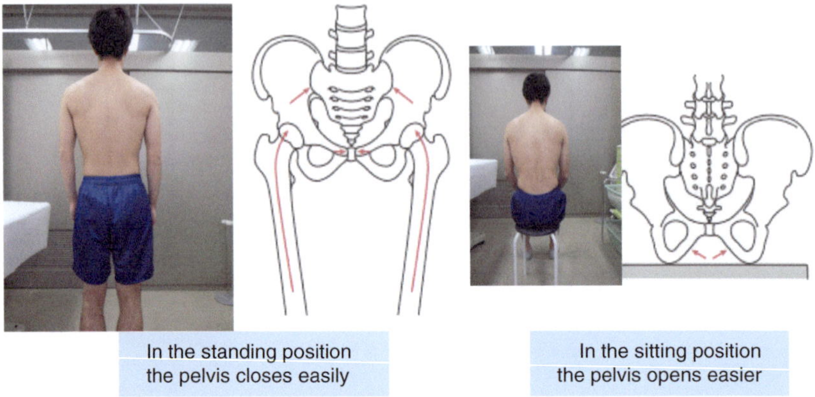

Fig. 3.3 Effect of standing position and sitting position on the pelvis. In the standing position, force is transmitted from the lower limbs to the hip bone and works in a direction which closes the SIJ. In the sitting position, the weight of the upper body is applied to the sciatic bone, making the pelvis open more easily. The female pelvis is especially easy to distort in the sitting position because the opening of the ischia is angled wide. So, the pelvis closes easily when standing and opens easily when sitting (Nobuko Watanabe: Nikkei BP company, Tokyo, p. 82, 2009)

3.1.2 Classification of SIJ Disorder (Fig. 3.4)

SIJ disorder is roughly classified into two categories. One is inflammation in the cavity, such as infection or seronegative spondyloarthropathy.

However these cases are rare. The other is joint dysfunction with minor joint subluxation which are the majority of SIJ disorder.

SIJ disorder is classified with Bernard's classification as a reference [6], as follows:

1. SIJ dysfunction: SIJ dysfunction is essentially minor subluxation of the joint and not inflammation. Hence, there are no specific findings in MRI or CT images.
2. Infection: Infections in the joint cavity are likely to show obvious abnormal findings on MRI.
3. Seronegative spondyloarthropathy (SNSA): including seven diseases (Table 3.1): These diseases are likely to complicate inflammation in the SIJ.
4. Degenerative arthritis: There are some cases in which pain is caused by arthrosis in the SIJ. Furthermore, cases of arthropathy which have no correlation with SIJ pain are not few.
5. Metabolism: Crystals can be deposited in the sacroiliac joints, due to gout, pseudogout, hyperparathyroidism, etc.

   There are some cases in which these cause inflammation.

Fig. 3.4 Two categories of SIJ disorder

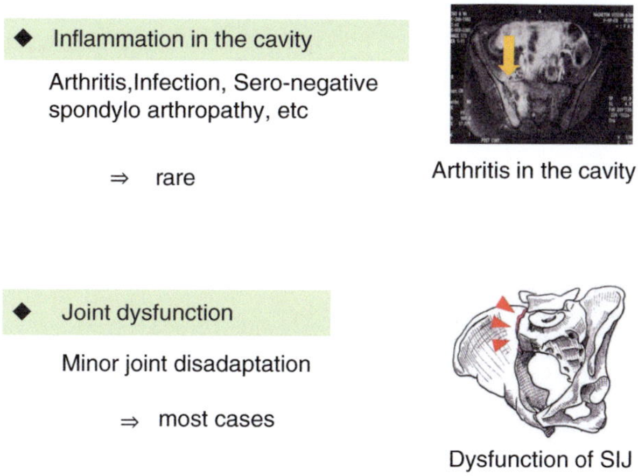

Table 3.1 Seronegative spondyloarthropathy (SNSA): consisting of seven diseases [22]

1. Ankylosing spondylitis: AS
Ankylosing spondylitis spreads mainly into the spine but can also found in peripheral joints. On an X-ray, a bamboo spine shadow is a typical finding
2. Psoriatic arthritis: PsA
Patients with psoriasis have complications from swelling and pain in their joints due to arthritis
3. Reiter syndrome: RS
Arthritis following urethritis and diarrhea is common for this disease. Three typical symptoms of the disease are arthritis, conjunctivitis, and urethritis
4. Crohn's disease
Fever, abdominal pain, and diarrhea are characteristic symptoms of this disease. Arthritis is a complication in 15% of patients with the disease. Inflamed granulated tissue is commonly found in the Iliocecal region
5. Ulcerative colitis
Mucinous bloody diarrhea is a characteristic symptom in this condition. Arthritis is a complication in 10% of patients with this disease. The colon, especially the rectum, is commonly diseased
6. Whipple disease
Abdominal pain and diarrhea are characteristics of this disease. Arthritis is a complication in many patients. The disease develops easily in the intestines
7. Behcet's disease
Lower right abdominal pain and bleeding are the major symptoms of this disease. Many patients have complications from arthritis. The disease develops easily in the ascending colon, the cecum, and the ending part of the ileum

6. Neoplastic: This is when a primary tumor of the sacrum/iliac bone or a metastatic tumor lesion extends to near the cartilage of the SIJ.
7. Traumatic: SIJ pain occurs due to a fatigue fracture of the sacrum or instability after a traumatic injury to the SIJ.

8. Iatrogenic: SIJ pain develops due to damage to the SIJ which occurred when obtaining bone tips for grafting. We treated several patients with SIJ pain that was most likely due to a ligament injury in the bone-muscle section of the SIJ.

Key Message: Dysfunction of the SIJ Resembles Minor Subluxation of the Elbow in a Child
Children sometimes have minor subluxation of the elbow, where the head of the radius becomes minutely subluxed and causes dysfunction. Dysfunction of the SIJ is similar to subluxation of the elbow in a child from a mechanical viewpoint. Both conditions show no findings on MRI or CT examination (Fig. 3.5).

3.1.3 The Prevalence of SIJ Disorder

In clinical reviews, the prevalence of SIJ disorder among patients with low back pain is 3.5–30%, [7–9].

From December 1999 to November 2000, the patients with SIJ disorder at our hospital were 54 out of 504 new patients with low back pain [10]. The prevalence of it was 11% (Table 3.2). Recently, attention has been payed to SIJ disorder which develops after fusion of lumbar vertebrae with instruments. Unoki et al. [11]

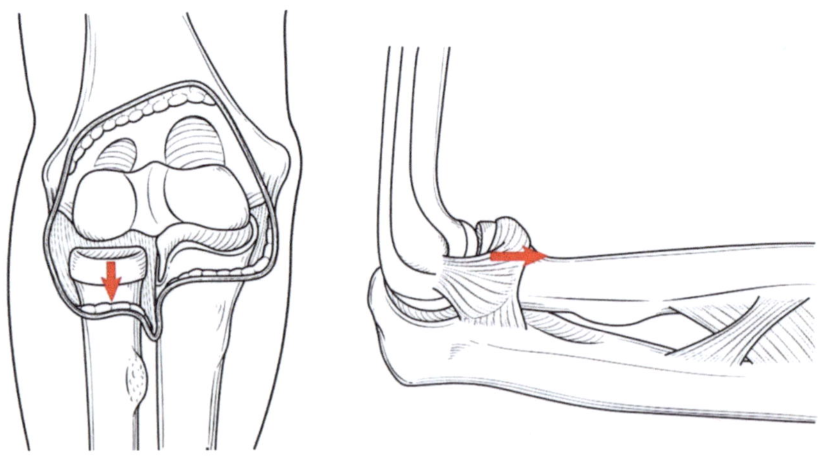

Fig. 3.5 Dysfunction of the SIJ resembles minor subluxation of the elbow in a child. Dysfunction of the SIJ is similar to subluxation of the elbow in a child, where the condition shows no findings on MRI or CT examination. With permission from [23]

Table 3.2 The prevalence of SIJ disorder among patients with low back pain (<75 years old)

New patients with low back pain	504
Patients with SIJ disorder…	54 (11%)

From December 1999 to November 2000 in our hospital

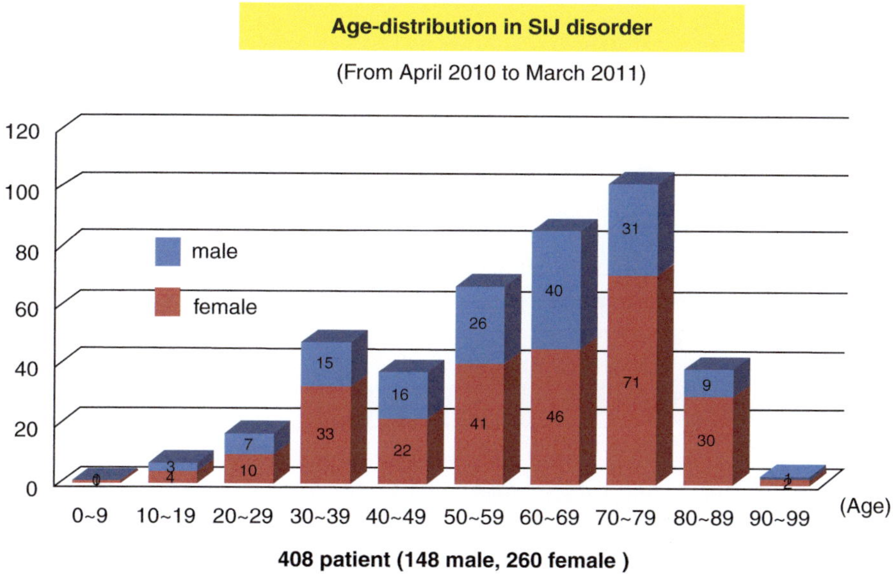

Fig. 3.6 Age distribution of patients with SIJ disorder. This graph shows that SIJ disorder is a common disease, occurring in people of all ages and both sexes

reported that SIJ disorder developed in 15% of the patients who underwent fusion of their lumbar vertebrae and the prevalence of the disorder in patients with fusion was more than in those without fusion.

3.1.4 Age Distribution

During 1 year in the Low Back Pain/Sacroiliac Joint Center, established in April 2010, we treated 408 patients that consisted of 148 males and 260 females. These patients were distributed over a wide age range between 9 and over 90 years old. Among them, the youngest patient was a 9-year-old girl. Our data shows that SIJ disorder is a common disease which causes low back pain and occurs in people of all ages and in both sexes (Fig. 3.6), despite SIJ disorder often being thought of as pain related to childbirth and specific to women.

3.1.5 Bilateral SIJ Pain

Bernard et al. [7] stated that pain developed bilaterally in 20% of patients with SIJ disorder. We have certainly treated some patients who had bilateral SIJ pain upon first consultation at our hospital. However, most of them initially had pain unilaterally; pain on the opposite side gradually developed.

3.1.6 Combination of SIJ Disorder and Lumbar Spinal Lesions

Bernard et al. [7] reported that SIJ disorder was associated with 23% of patients with low back pain. Cases in which there is a combination of lumbar spinal lesions and SIJ disorder are not few. Some cases become complicated with SIJ disorder soon after surgery for lumbar spinal lesions.

In order to confirm which is the main condition, we should look for any change in symptoms, while making full use of nerve root blocks and SIJ injections. Based on the response to the injections, we can suppose a rough ratio of the conditions, like "40% lumbar spinal lesion + 60% SIJ disorder," "70% lumbar spinal lesion + 30% SIJ disorder," etc.

It is important to recognize that patients who have a combination of lumbar disease and SIJ disorder are not few. Lacking this recognition may lead you to misdiagnose and perform unnecessary surgery on the patient.

3.2 Clinical Features

3.2.1 Pain Areas of SIJ Disorder

As some studies have indicated, pain due to SIJ disorder spreads over the gluteal, posterior thigh areas and down to the ankle [12], as well as from the low abdominal area to the groin [13]. In our study, 94 of 100 patients reported *pain at or around the posterior-superior iliac spine (PSIS)*. Leg symptoms of SIJ disorder comprised pain and a numbness/tingling sensation, and ≥60% of the patients had these symptoms. Pain was mainly detected in the back, buttock, *groin*, and thigh areas (Fig. 3.7a), while numbness/tingling was mainly detected in the lateral to posterior thigh and back of the calf, not in the gluteal or groin areas (Fig. 3.7b). *Leg symptoms do not usually correspond to the dermatome of lumbar nerve roots* [14].

Considering the nerve distribution to SIJ, there is a possibility that SIJ disorder may cause pain in various areas as lower lumbar nerve roots and sacral nerve roots distribute rami to the SIJ. However, in actuality most SIJ disorders have specific pain areas. Hence, paying attention to these pain areas can help us differentiate patients with SIJ disorder from those with lumbar disc herniation or lumbar spinal stenosis.

When we inject hypertonic saline into the SIJ, in most cases *gluteal pain at or around the PSIS* initially develops, and so it is supposed that *this area is specific to SIJ disorder* (Fig. 3.8). Some cases cause leg symptoms which cannot be distinguished from femoral neuralgia or sciatica.

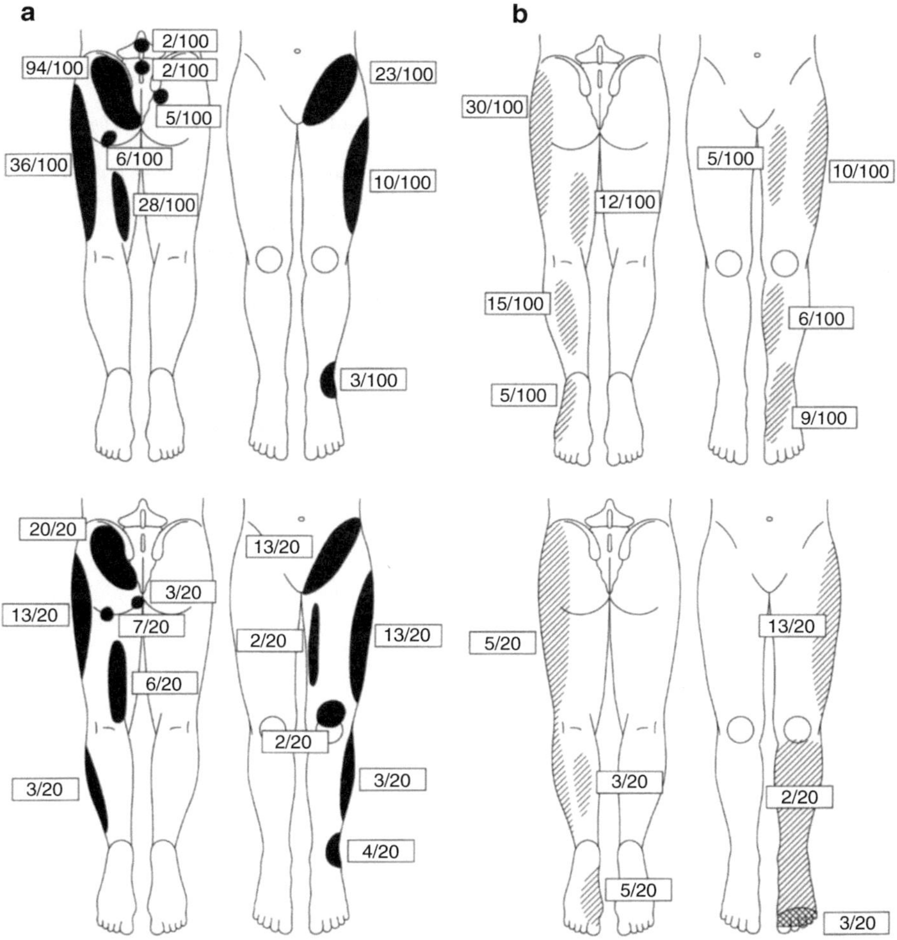

Fig. 3.7 Clinical features of SIJ disorder. The upper figure represents a group of 100 cases of SIJ disorder treated with conservative therapy. The lower figure represents a group of 20 cases of severe SIJ disorder treated with SIJ fusion. (**a**) Pain was mainly detected in the proximal leg, such as the gluteal, groin, and thigh areas. (**b**) Numbness was mainly detected in the distal leg, not in the gluteal

Until now, attention has been paid only to leg pain which corresponds to the dermatome of lumbar nerve roots for surgery. However, symptoms which do not correspond to the dermatome of lumbar nerve roots are actually not uncommon. It is necessary to accurately detect symptoms in order to correctly diagnose a disease.

3.2.2 Differentiation Between Leg Symptoms from SIJ Disorder and Those from Damaged Lumbar Roots

If you observe leg symptoms which do not usually correspond to the dermatome of lumbar nerve roots, you should suspect referred pain from ligaments or joints. Additionally, when careful attention is paid to leg symptoms, you will discover that

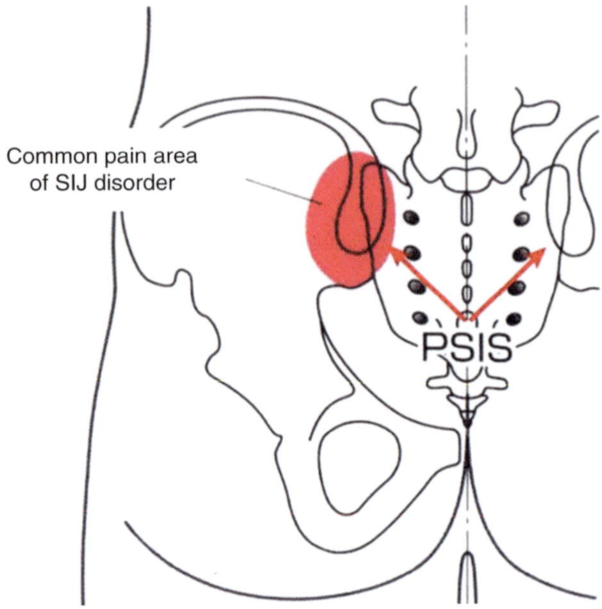

Fig. 3.8 Specific pain area of SIJ disorder. Injecting hypertonic saline into the SIJ initially induces gluteal pain around the PSIS in most cases. With permission from [23]

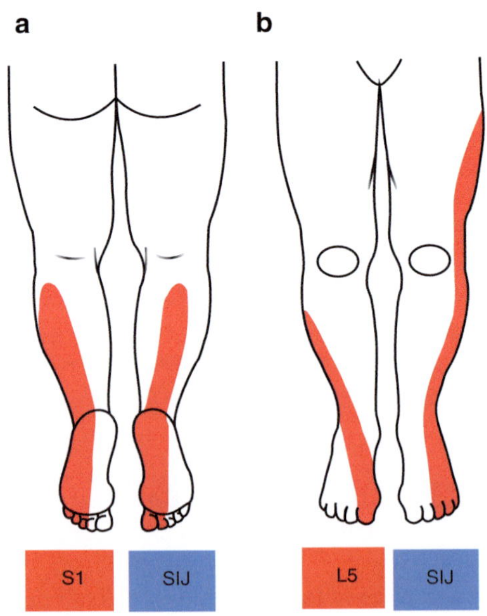

Fig. 3.9 Differentiation between leg symptoms of SIJ disorder and those of L5, S1 damaged lumbar roots. With permission from [23]. (**a**) S1 root/SIJ disorder. S1 root: pain or numbness from the calf to the lateral foot. SIJ disorder: occasional pain or numbness from the calf to the medial foot. (**b**) L5 root/SIJ disorder. L5 root: pain or numbness from the lateral leg to the medial foot. SIJ disorder: occasional pain or numbness from the lateral thigh and leg to the lateral foot

referred pain areas from ligaments are different from those caused by damaged lumbar nerve roots.

The S1 root usually causes pain or numbness from the calf to the lateral foot. On the other hand, SIJ disorder sometimes causes pain or numbness from the calf to the medial foot. Furthermore, the L5 root usually causes pain or numbness from the lateral leg to the medial foot, whereas SIJ disorder can cause pain or numbness from the lateral thigh and leg to the lateral foot (Fig. 3.9a, b).

Careful attention to leg symptoms enables us to understand whether the symptoms are caused by damaged lumbar roots or referred pain from diseases such as SIJ disorder.

Key Message: Entire Lateral Thigh Pain Is Not Derived from Damaged Lumbar Roots

If pain is observed in the entire lateral thigh, from the great trochanter to the lateral knee, first suspect pain derived from SIJ disorder.

In our study, we compared pain in the lateral thigh from lumbar nerve roots with that from SIJ disorder. Pain areas of totally 32 nerve roots that included L2, L3, L4, L5, and S1 nerve roots were examined. Lateral thigh pain involving the great trochanter was found only in one damaged L2 root and one damaged L3 root. However, lateral thigh pain from the great trochanter to the lateral knee was not found in the stimulated lumbar nerve roots. On the other hand, 5 of 10 patients with SIJ disorder had pain at the lateral thigh (Fig. 3.10).

Regarding lateral thigh pain, entire lateral thigh pain from the great trochanter to the lateral knee is not derived from damaged lumbar roots, but SIJ disorder often causes pain in this area (Fig. 3.11). Careful attention to pain in the lateral thigh enables us to understand whether the symptoms are derived from damaged lumbar roots or referred pains from such as SIJ disorder.

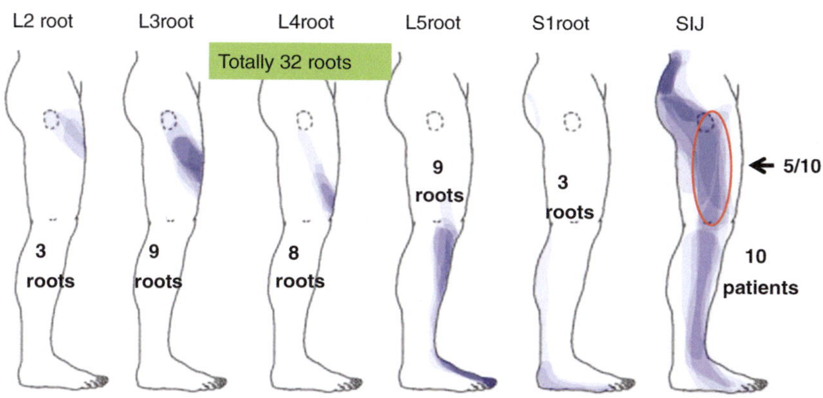

Fig. 3.10 Pain in the lateral thigh. Pain areas of 32 total nerve roots, that included L2, L3, L4, L5, and S1 nerve roots, were examined. Lateral thigh pain from the great trochanter to the lateral knee was not caused when stimulating lumbar nerve roots, while patients with SIJ disorder had pain in that area in five out of ten cases

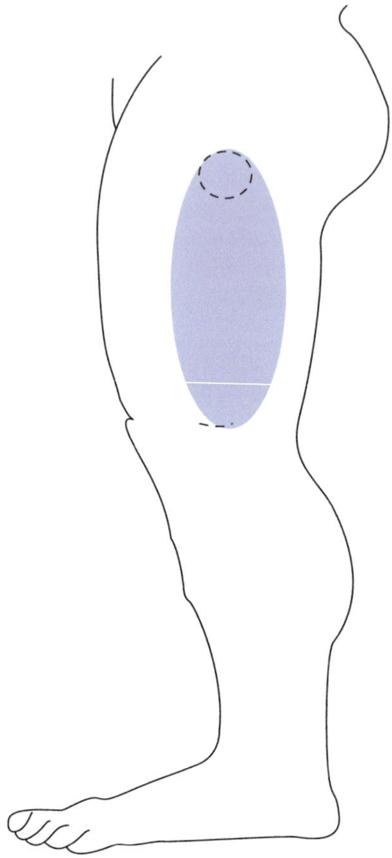

Fig. 3.11 Entire lateral thigh pain. Pain in the entire lateral thigh is not thought to be derived from damaged lumbar nerve roots, but SIJ disorder often causes pain in the area

3.2.3 Characteristic Motions and Postures Which Induce SIJ Pain

First, patients with SIJ disorder have pain when sitting on a chair.

Second, the patients have pain when in a supine position or lying on their side, especially on the affected side. Furthermore, pain develops when turning over in bed, standing up from a chair, and early in the morning, which are characteristic of joint pain (Table 3.3). In addition, some people complained of pain in the perineal area when urinating or evacuating.

In a supine position, pain can occur due to the distorting of the SIJ by the load created by a patient's own weight.

In some severe cases, patients cannot sit, walk, or lie in a supine position. It is not uncommon that their pain can only be easily relieved in the prone position.

Table 3.3 Motion-related pain relieved after joint arthrodesis (in 15 patients with arthrodesis)

Pain in a supine position: 15
Pain when lying on their side: 14
Pain when sitting on a chair: 13
Pain when walking: 8
Pain when standing: 7
Pain when sitting on the patient's heels with a straight back: 2

In most patients with severe pain, requiring arthrodesis, pain in a supine position, while lying on their side or sitting on a chair, was relieved after surgery. Before surgery, patients rarely had pain when sitting on the their heels with a straight back

Especially, it is specific to SIJ disorder that patients feel pain when sitting on a hard chair. We have experienced cases where patients undergo examination while raising their affected buttock off the chair to prevent developing pain. We think that the length of time to be able to sit on a chair should be useful in evaluating the extent to which patients have recovered from the disease.

3.2.4 Discrimination of Pain Area in Sitting Between Lumbar Lesions and SIJ Disorder

In our data [15], the prevalence of pain caused by a sitting position was 73% for SIJ disorder, 49% for lumbar disc herniation, and 20% for lumbar spinal canal stenosis. Moreover, pain from SIJ disorder when sitting was found close to the PSIS and in the ischial tuberosity. On the other hand, in cases of hernia or stenosis, pain developed in the center of the gluteal region and in the region of femoral neuralgia and sciatica. Thus, the prevalence of pain from SIJ disorder when sitting is higher than that of lumbar disc herniation and lumbar spinal canal stenosis. As well, the pain areas associated with SIJ disorder are different from those caused by lumbar lesions. Hence, in many cases SIJ disorder can be differentiated from lumbar lesions.

Key Message: Principle of Pain Provocation in Sitting: Fixing the Ischial Tuberosity Induces Distortion in the SIJ

In the sitting position, as the ischial tuberosity is fixed on the seat, distortion in the SIJ occurs and pain develops (Fig. 3.12).

On the other hand, pain is not so induced in sitting on their heels, because the ischial tuberosity is not fixed. Work in sitting is necessary on daily life and so, this is a large problem in modern civilized age.

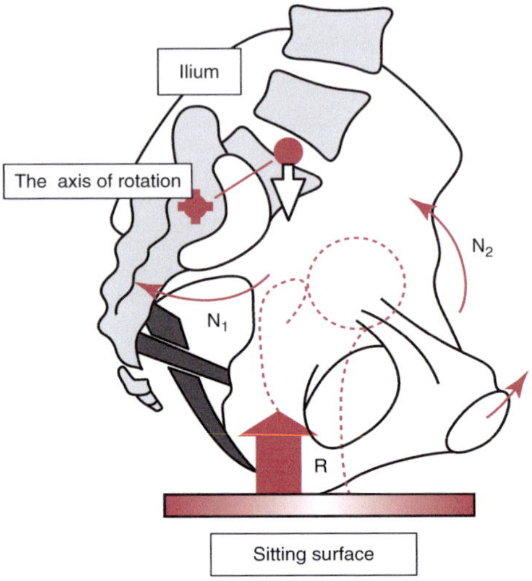

Fig. 3.12 Principle of pain provocation in sitting. Fixing the ischial tuberosity induces distortion in the SIJ and pain can develop. With permission from [23]. *P* body weight, *R* repulsion power, *N1* posterior rotational moment, *N2* anterior rotational moment

3.3 Physical Findings

3.3.1 Neurological Findings

SIJ disorder does not usually show a neurological deficit. However, some patients have symptoms resembling muscle weakness at first glance and complain that they cannot extend their lower limbs forward, and as a result they fall down.

It seems that this condition is due to a loss of muscular tonus developing at the moment when a load is added (See Table 2.2).

Some patients complain of being unable to feel the brake of their car as they step on it due to severe SIJ disorder. In severe cases, they complain of certain symptoms, a lack of sense of position, and obvious sensory disturbances, which do not correspond to the dermatome of lumbar nerve roots.

3.3.2 Tenderness Points

We [16] compared the prevalence of tenderness on the nine points of pelvic girdle (the PSIS, the long posterior sacroiliac ligament, the gluteal muscle, the superior gluteal nerve, the sacrotuberous ligament, the piriformis muscle, the iliac muscle, the Scarpa triangle, and the pubic syndesmosis among patients with SIJ disorder and those with lumbar lesions. Out of nine tenderness points, the PSIS, the long posterior sacroiliac ligament, the sacrotuberous ligament, and the iliac muscle were specific to SIJ disorder. The sensitivity and specificity of these tenderness points were examined as follows: the PSIS (53%, 85%), the long posterior sacroiliac ligament (60%, 84%), the sacrotuberous ligament (40%, 86%), and the iliac muscles (71%, 71%) were significantly higher than in patients with lumbar lesions (Fig. 3.13).

We place emphasis on these tenderness points. We believe that these points help us in diagnosing SIJ disorder.

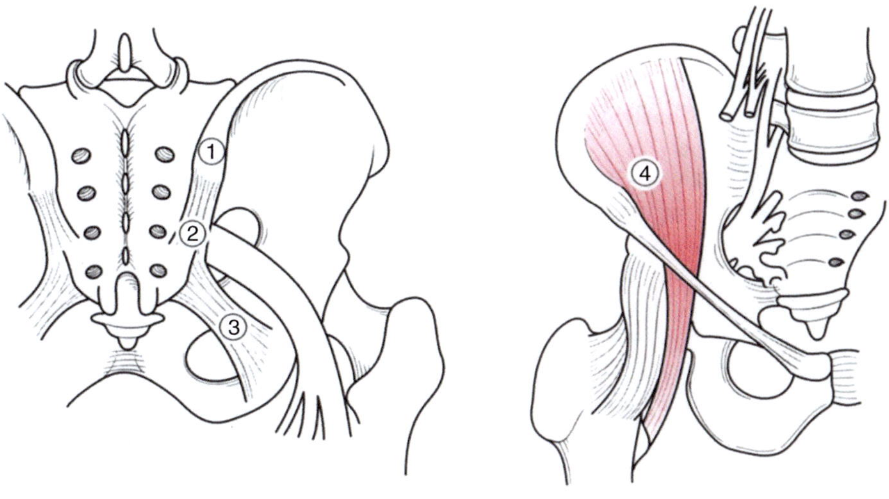

Fig. 3.13 The characteristic points of tenderness in SIJ disorder. Tenderness on the PSIS (**1**), the long posterior sacroiliac ligament (**2**), the sacrotuberous ligament (**3**), and the iliac muscle (**4**) are specific to SIJ disorder

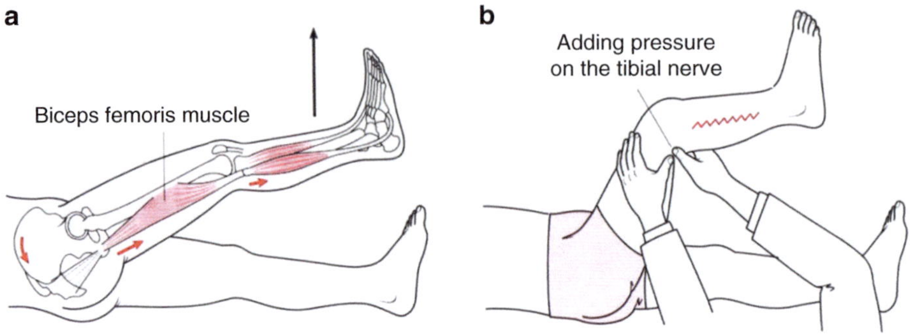

Fig. 3.14 The bowstring sign maneuver differentiates SIJ disorder from LDH. With permission from [23]. (**a**) The SLR test: This is a useful test which induces symptoms of compressed lumbar nerve roots (sciatica) in LDH. However, this test can also induce SIJ pain due to the backward rotation of the ilium by the pulling of the biceps femoris muscle tendon, which attaches to the ischial tuberosity. (**b**) The bowstring sign maneuver: As the bowstring sign maneuver cannot easily induce SIJ pain, this maneuver should be considered useful for differentiating sciatica from SIJ disorder

3.3.3 Difference Between the Straight Leg Raising (SLR) Test and the BowString Sign

In general, the SLR is used as a useful test which induces symptoms of compressed lumbar nerve roots, such as in lumbar disc herniation (Fig. 3.14a). It is thought that the test induces sciatica by tightening the roots compressed by lumbar disc herniation. However, SIJ pain can also be induced by the SLR test. The assumed mechanism of this test is that the pulling of the biceps femoris muscle tendon, which attaches to the ischial tuberosity, followed by a rotation backward of the ilium, causes SIJ pain.

In addition, when pushing the tibial nerve using your thumb on the popliteal area at an angle where the SLR test induces pain, while bending the patient's knee, sciatica can be reproduced. This is called the bowstring sign (Fig. 3.14b).

This maneuver does not pull the tendon of the biceps femoris muscle and therefore the ilium does not rotate. SIJ pain should not easily occur from this test. The bowstring sign maneuver should be considered useful for discriminating sciatica from SIJ pain.

3.4 Findings from Image and Blood Examinations

3.4.1 Image Findings

Using the current imaging methods, no findings which are useful for diagnosing SIJ disorder can be detected (Table 3.4).

Table 3.4 Imaging methods: findings useful in diagnosing SIJ disorder have not been detected

1. X-ray
X-ray does not always indicate a finding for current SIJ pain
2. CT
There is not a strong relationship between changes in the SIJ and SIJ pain
3. MRI
MRI is very useful for diagnosing pyogenic sacroiliac arthritis and neoplastic changes. However, the diagnostic value for SIJ pain is unknown
4. Bone scintigram
The degree of specificity of the disease by bone scintigraphy is low

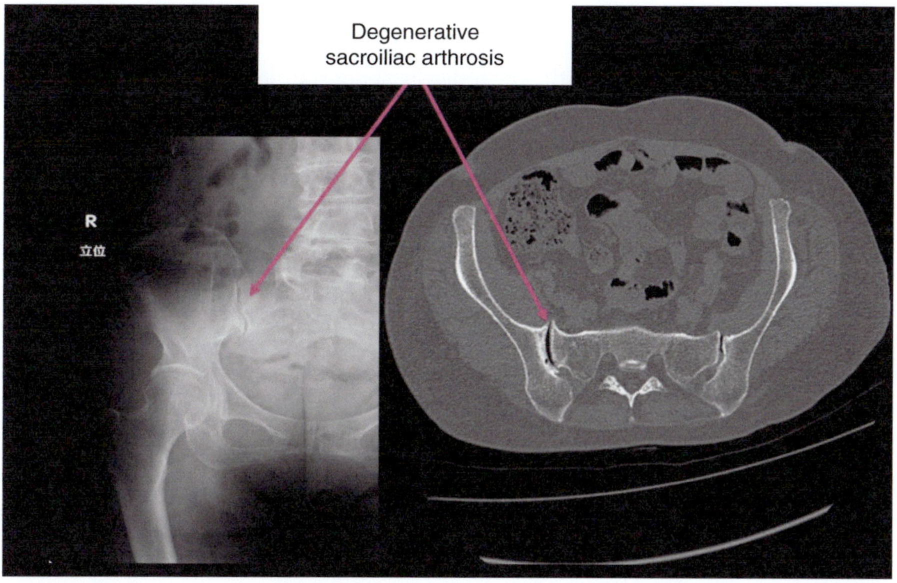

Fig. 3.15 Degenerative sacroiliac arthrosis. With permission from [23]. Bony spurs and sclerotic changes on the edge of the joint should be found

3.4.1.1 X-ray Findings

Saito et al. [17] examined the relationship between osteosclerosis of the SIJ and SIJ pain, in patients with unilateral hip osteoarthritis. As a result, on the side with hip osteoarthritis, osteosclerosis of the SIJ was seen in approximately 57% of patients, but SIJ pain was seen in only 20%. He reported that there was no significant relationship between osteosclerosis of the SIJ and SIJ pain.

Moreover, SIJ pain likely developed on the side with hip osteoarthritis, and SIJ osteosclerosis tended to occur on the healthy side of the hip joint. Osteosclerosis of the SIJ suggests that the SIJ has born a heavy load in the past. It does not always indicate a finding that the SIJ is the cause of the current pain (Fig. 3.15).

3.4.1.2 CT Findings

It is thought that there isn't a strong relationship between changes in the joint and pain, though CT is effective to know any changes in bones and joint space [6].

3.4.1.3 MRI Findings

MRI is very useful for diagnosing pyogenic sacroiliac arthritis, neoplastic changes around the joints, and osteoporotic fractures. The diagnostic value for SIJ pain is unknown [6].

3.4.1.4 Bone Scintigraphic Findings

The specificity of disease by bone scintigraphic method is low because accumulation images are found not only in regions with inflammation and neoplastic lesions but also in those with bone fractures and arthropathy [6].

As described above, it is difficult to detect abnormal finding in SIJ dysfunction using the current imaging methods. In order to diagnose SIJ disorder, the investigation of a medical history, symptoms, and physical findings is important. Furthermore, it is necessary to recognize that the image findings do not directly indicate the disease. Even if the ability of diagnostic imaging devices improves in the future, it is necessary to accurately examine whether the image findings indicate symptoms or not.

3.4.2 Recent Topics Surrounding Image Findings

3.4.2.1 SPECT/CT Findings

Recently, it has been revealed that some patients with chronic severe SIJ disorder have high-uptake finding on SPECT/CT [18] (Fig. 3.16).

3.4.2.2 Ultrasound Findings

There are some patients with chronic SIJ disorder who show irregular tissue in the posterior sacroiliac ligaments under ultrasound (Fig. 3.17).

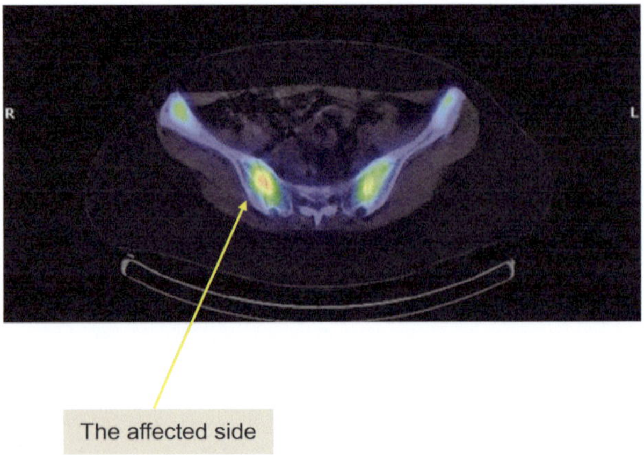

Fig. 3.16 Findings on SPECT/CT. High-uptake finding on SPECT/CT is shown on the affected side

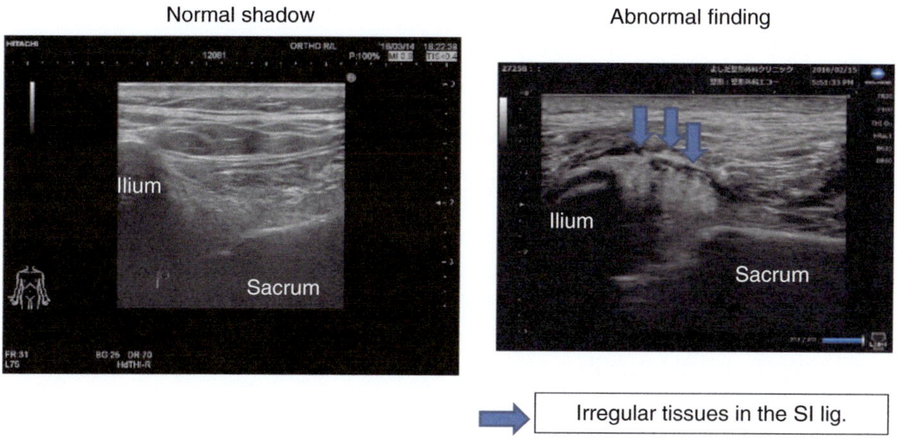

Fig. 3.17 Ultrasound findings. From Shinichi Yoshida

3.4.3 Findings from Blood Investigation

SIJ disorder is basically dysfunction due to minor subluxation of the joint. There is the possibility that a local micro-inflammation will develop due to SIJ disorder. However, a whole body inflammation, where abnormal counts of C-reactive protein (CRP) and white blood cells (WBC) are detected, is not usually observed. Blood test findings useful for diagnosing other diseases are shown in Table 3.5.

Table 3.5 Blood test findings useful for diagnosis of other diseases

1. Pyogenic spondylitis
The patient has fever and back pain as well as an increase in WBC and CRP
2. Periodic tetraplegia
An abnormality in the serum potassium level causes flaccid paralysis (bilateral symmetry) of the skeletal muscles. A low serum potassium level is often caused by hyperthyroidism and aldosteronism
3. Diabetic peripheral neuropathy
This is a form of polyneuropathy which exhibits an abnormal sensation in the distal area of the limbs. It is described as "glove and sock peripheral neuropathy." Abnormally high levels of Hb A1c and blood glucose can be detected
4. Metastatic bone tumor
There is an elevation of ALP in the blood
5. Bleeding tendency
Blood diseases, liver dysfunction, and drug use can cause thrombocytopenia and dysfunction in coagulation

Key Message: Iliosclerotic Ostitis and Degenerative Sacroiliac Arthropathy

Iliosclerotic ostitis has a triangular osteosclerotic shadow on an X-ray, which is localized at the lower part of the iliac bone that is in contact with the SIJ. However, this indicates a finding of non-specific ischemic change, which is not inflammatory (Fig. 3.18). Iliosclerotic ostitis is likely to occur in women who have experienced childbirth. This finding is considered to be a reactive change after a load has been put on the pelvis. The percentage of iliosclerotic ostitis was 1.4% in examinations of healthy people, and all cases with abnormality were woman [19]. It is thought that this finding is not directly related to SIJ pain.

This disease can be distinguished from arthropathy, which has osteophyte formations around the SIJ and develops in elderly men and women, by the shadow on an X-ray.

Key Message: Asymptomatic MRI Findings

The existence of asymptomatic MRI findings has been known. It has been reported that 57% of asymptomatic people over 60 years old had some abnormality in their lumbar MRI [20]. A survey of lumbar MRI results also indicated that there was not much difference in the frequency of abnormal intervertebral discs between people with low back pain and those without pain [21].

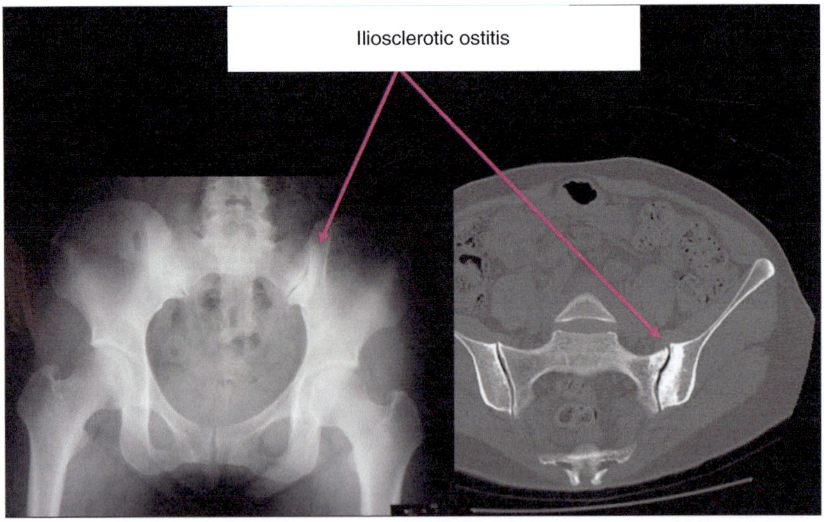

Fig. 3.18 Iliosclerotic ostitis. Having a triangular osteosclerotic shadow localized at the lower part of the iliac bone is characteristic. This shadow does not indicate a finding of SIJ disorder, but non-specific ischemic change. With permission from [23]

References

1. MacConaill MA, Basmajian JV. Muscles and Movements – a basis for human kinesiology, vol. 60. Baltimore: Williams and Wilkins; 1969.
2. Borowsky CD, Fagen G. Sources of sacroiliac region pain: insights gained from a study comparing standard intra-articular injection with a technique combining intra-and periarticular injection. Arch Phys Med Rehabil. 2008;89:2048–56.
3. Murakami E, Tanaka Y, Aizawa T, et al. Effect of peri-articular and intra-articular injections for sacroiliac joint pain: a prospective comparative study. J Orthop Sci. 2007;12:274–80.
4. Yoshida K. Structural medical science: Shizenchiyu no kagi wa juryoku ni aru. Enterprise: Tokyo; 1999. p. 148–52. (in Japanese).
5. Kapandgi IA. The physiology of the joints, vol. 3. The trunk and the vertebral column. Edinburgh: Churchill Livingstone; 1974.
6. Bernard TN Jr, Cassidy JD. The sacroiliac joint syndrome: pathophysiology, diagnosis, and management. In: Frymoyer JW, editor. The adult spine: principles and practice. New York: Raven Press; 1991. p. 2107–30.
7. Bernard TN, Kirkaldy-Willis WH. Recognizing specific characteristics of nonspecific low back pain. Clin Orthop Relat Res. 1987;217:266–80.
8. Solonen KA. The sacroiliac joint in the light of anatomical, roentgen logical and clinical studies. Acta Orthop Scand Suppl. 1957;27:1–127.
9. Schwarzer AC, Aprill CN, Bogduk N. The sacroiliac joint in chronic low back pain. Spine. 1995;20:31–7.
10. Murakami E, Kanno H, Kokubun S, Tanaka Y. Sacroiliac joint pain: any tenderness points can indicate a patient with the pain? J Jpn Spine Res Soc. 2002;13:24. (in Japanese).
11. Unoki E, Abe E, Murai H, et al. Fusion of multiple segments can increase the incidence of sacroiliac joint pain after lumbar or lumbosacral fusion. Spine. 2016;41:999–1005.
12. Kirkaldy-Willis WH. The site and nature of the lesion. Managing low back pain. New York: Churchill Livingstone; 1983. p. 91–107.
13. Norman GF. Sacroiliac disease and its relationship to lower abdominal pain. Am J Surg. 1968;116:54–6.
14. Murakami E, Aizawa T, Kurosawa D. Leg symptoms associated with sacroiliac joint disorder and related pain. Clin Neurol Neurosurg. 2017;157:55–8.
15. Kawakami J, Kurosawa D, Murakami E. Pain areas by sitting originated from sacroiliac joint dysfunction are different from those from lumbar disorders. Seikeigeka. 2014;65:513–7. (in Japanese).
16. Kurosawa D, Murakami E. Pelvic girdle tenderness points to differentiate the sacroiliac joint dysfunction from lumbar diseases. Seikeigeka. 2012;63:1231–5. (in Japanese).
17. Saito A, Kikuchi S, Yabuki S, Takeda K. The influence of the coxarthrosis to the sacroiliac joint. Clin Orthop Surg. 2002;37:231–6. (in Japanese).
18. Tofuku K, Koga H, Komiya S. The diagnostic value of single-photon emission computed tomography/computed tomography for severe sacroiliac joint dysfunction. Eur Spine J. 2015;24:859–63.
19. Kikuchi S. Youtsu (Bachache). Tokyo: Igaku-Syoin; 2003. p. 181–5. (in Japanese).
20. Boden SD, Davis DO, Dina TS, et al. Abnormal magnetic-resonance scans of the lumbar spine in asymptomatic subjects. A prospective investigation. J Bone Joint Surg Am. 1990;72:403–8.
21. Boos N, Rieder R, Schade V, et al. The diagnostic accuracy of magnetic resonance imaging, work perception, and psychosocial factors in identifying symptomatic disc herniations. Spine. 1995;20:2613–25.
22. Maruo S, editor. Seikeigeka shinryo memo. 3rd ed. Tokyo: Nankodo; 2003. p. 106. (in Japanese).
23. Murakami E. Sacroiliac joint pain: undiagnosed low back pain. Tokyo: Nankodo; 2012. (in Japanese).

4 Diagnosis of Sacroiliac Joint Disorder

Abstract

- Pain at or around the PSIS, groin pain, and pain at or around the ischial tuberosity are characteristic of SIJ disorder.
- The one-finger test is useful for identifying pain areas. Eighty-five percent of patients who indicate pain at or around the PSIS using the one-finger test are those with SIJ disorder.
- A peri-articular injection is easier to perform than an intra-articular injection. In about 80% of patients with SIJ disorder, peri-articular injection is effective.
- First a peri-articular injection should be performed, and, if ineffective, an intra-articular injection should be done for diagnosing SIJ disorder. Using this algorithm more SIJ pain will be diagnosed.
- A diagnostic scoring system is useful to differenciate between SIJ disorder and lumbar lesions.

4.1 Characteristic Pain Areas of SIJ Disorder

Gluteal pain at or around the PSIS, groin pain, and pain around the ischial tuberosity are characteristic of SIJ disorder, when compared to pain areas caused by lumbar disc herniation and lumbar spinal stenosis (Fig. 4.1) [1].

Paying attention to these pain areas can help us differentiate patients with SIJ disorder from those with lumbar disc herniation and lumbar spinal stenosis. Furthermore, many patients have thigh and leg pain and numbness, which do not correspond to the dermatome of lumbar nerve roots.

E. Murakami, *Sacroiliac Joint Disorder*,
https://doi.org/10.1007/978-981-13-1807-8_4

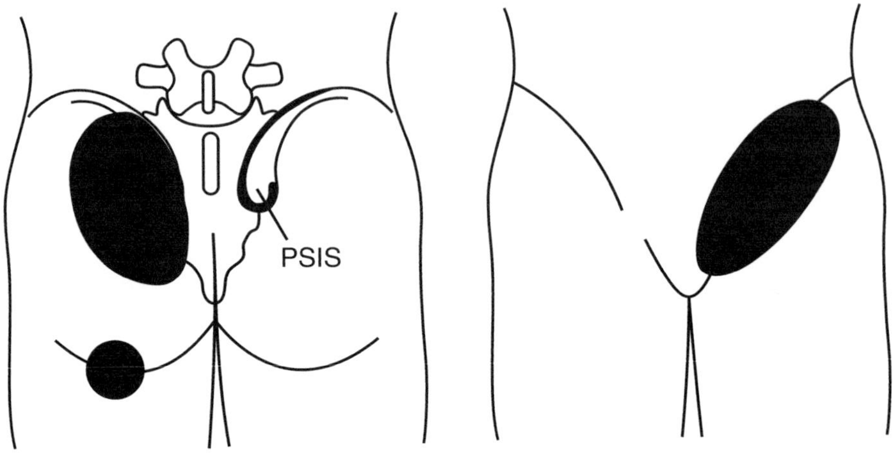

Fig. 4.1 Gluteal pain at or around the PSIS, groin pain, and pain around the ischial tuberosity are characteristic of SIJ disorder

Key Message: Do Not Be Deceived by Image Findings!
You should not give a wrong diagnosis based on MRI finding.

Lumbar disc herniation can be recognized on MRI (Fig. 4.2a), but the pain has been relieved after SIJ injections. Consequently, there is a possibility that symptoms could not get relieved, despite this case receiving a surgery for lumbar disc herniation. It is necessary to carefully examine whether or not a finding on MRI actually indicates the source of pain. With progress of imaging equipment in recent years, it is likely believed that all spinal diseases can be diagnosed by imaging. We should bear in mind that there are many patients with low back pain who cannot be diagnosed by the image.

Even if the ability of the image device improves in the future, a fundamental rule in detecting the origin of pain as follows will not change, forever. First you exclude the placebo response of the injection itself; it is necessary that the usual pain is reproduced by needle irritation or when injecting a local anesthetic with pressure. And then, pain is relieved by injection of a local anesthetic (Fig. 4.2b).

4.2 Examination

4.2.1 Pain Provocation Test

Many pain provocation tests for diagnosing SIJ disorder have been developed. However, it is thought that they do not have high specificity for the diagnosis of SIJ disorder alone [2]. Berthelot et al. [3] published a review article entitled "Provocative

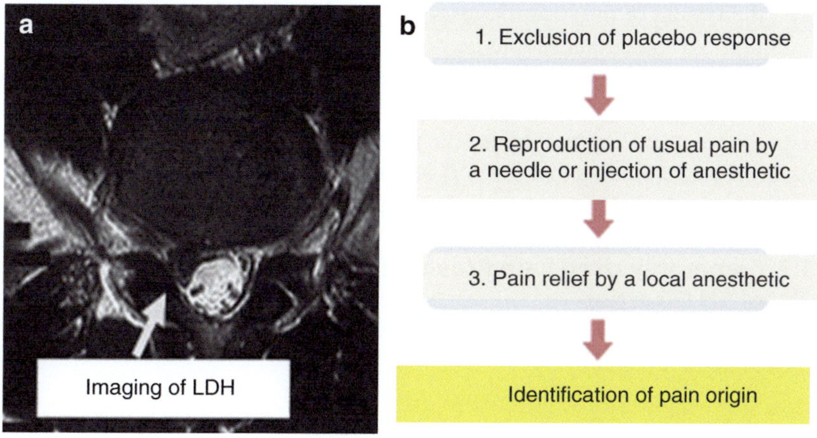

Fig. 4.2 (**a**) Clear image of a lumbar disc herniation. (**b**) Principle for the identification of the pain origin. With permission from [28]

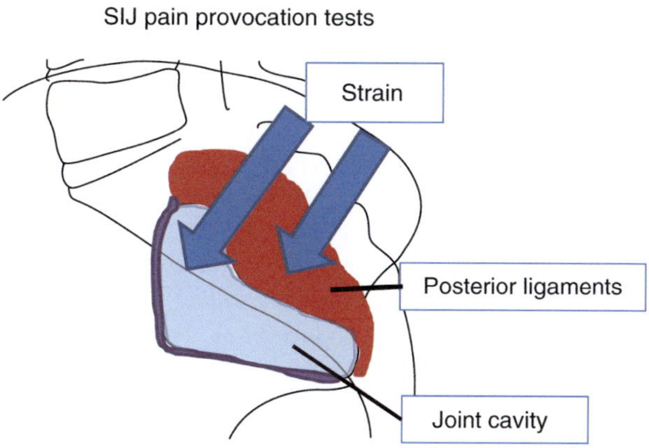

Fig. 4.3 SIJ pain provocation tests cause a strain on both the joint cavity and posterior ligaments

Sacroiliac Maneuvers and Sacroiliac Joint Block Are Unreliable for Diagnosing Sacroiliac Joint Pain."

4.2.1.1 Why Are Provocation Tests and SIJ Injections Unreliable?

The main reason for this is considered to be as follows: all regions of the joint structure can cause SIJ pain, including the joint cavity and posterior ligaments as stated in Chap. 2. As Kim et al. [4] reported, SIJ pain provocation tests could always cause a strain not only on the joint cavity but also on the posterior ligaments, due to a little motion of the joint (Fig. 4.3). Therefore, pain provocation tests can induce pain from not only the intra-articular region but also the peri-articular region. However, for the diagnosis of SIJ disorder, intra-articular injections, which will not anesthetize the peri-articular region, have been used. As a result, there is dissociation between the results of provocation tests and those of SIJ injection. Both intra- and peri-articular SIJ injections should be done for definitive diagnosis of SIJ disorder. If so, SIJ pain provocation tests and SIJ injections would provide substantial reliability for diagnosis.

Actually, we more commonly use the peri-articular injection for the diagnosis of SIJ disorder, based on data that the peri-articular injection is more effective than the intra-articular injection in most patients with SIJ disorder.

4.2.1.2 Commonly Used Pain Provocation Tests for the Assessment of SIJ Disorder

Laslett et al. argued that the combination of a few provocation tests was useful to detect SIJ disorder [5].

Gaenslen's Test (Fig. 4.4)

The patient lies supine near the edge of the table. One leg hangs over the edge of the table, and the other hip and knee are flexed toward the patient's chest. The examiner applies firm pressure to the knee being flexed toward the patient's chest while adding a counterpressure to the knee in the hanging leg. Positive test produces pain over the posterior SIJ on the side of hip joint extended. However, this test is little troublesome in the point that it has to be carried out after moving the patient near the edge of the table.

Patrick's Test (Fig. 4.4)

This test is also called as FABER (flexion, abduction, and external rotation) test. With the patient supine, this test is performed by flexion, abduction, and external rotation of the hip while pushing the knee of the evaluated side posteriorly; this maneuver stresses the hip and sacroiliac joint simultaneously. Positive test is commonly determined to reproduce back, buttock, or groin pain. Especially it is valuable to assess SIJ disorder when inducing pain over the posterior of the SIJ.

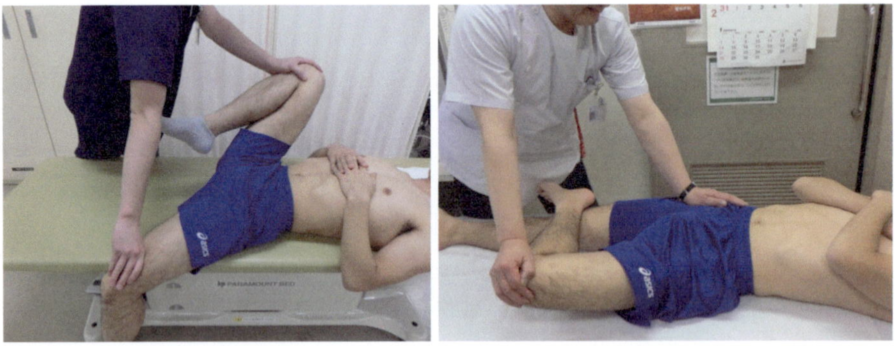

Gaenslen's test Patrick's test

Fig. 4.4 Gaenslen's test and Patrick's test

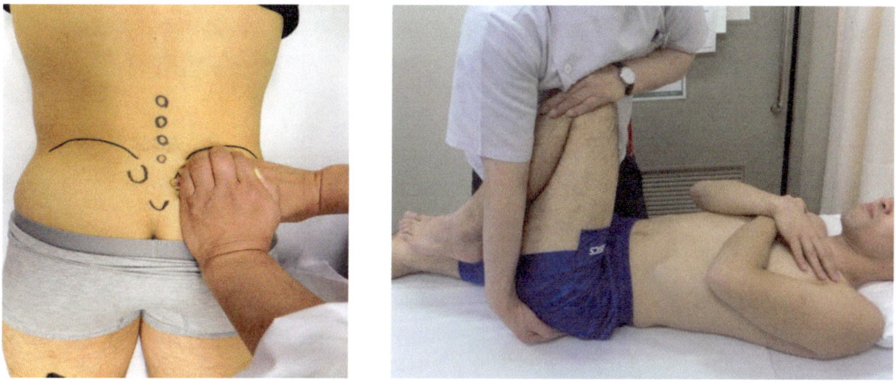

Sacroiliac joint shear test   Thigh thrust test

Fig. 4.5 Sacroiliac joint shear test and thigh thrust test

Sacroiliac Joint Shear Test (Fig. 4.5)
With a patient prone, the examiner places the palm of the hand over the posterior iliac wing and applies a force vertically downward, which produces a shearing force across the SIJ. Positive test reproduces familiar pain in a symptomatic SIJ. This test is the direct procedure to detect disorder of the SIJ, in which the SIJ is directly distorted, not through the femur as a lever arm. Furthermore, as the test with a patient prone can be easily carried out, successively following investigation of lumbar area, we generally use this test to detect SIJ disorder.

Thigh Thrust Test (Fig. 4.5)
The patient lies supine with the hip flexed where the thigh is at right angles to the table and then slightly adducted. The axial pressure is applied dorsally along the line of the femur. This test uses the femur as a lever to push the ilium posteriorly and is presumed to occur a posterior shearing force to the SIJ. Positive test reproduces familiar pain in a symptomatic SIJ. We consider that this test is also very useful to detect SIJ disorder.

Pelvic Distraction Test (Fig. 4.6)
With the patient supine, this test is performed by palpating the medial aspect of the ASIS bilaterally with the palms of the crossed hands. Apply a slow, steady, posterolateral force through the ASIS. Maintain the force for 5 s. Positive test reproduces familiar pain in a symptomatic SIJ.

Pelvic Compression Test (Fig. 4.6)
With the patient lying on the side with hips and knees moderately flexed, palpate the anterolateral aspect of the uppermost iliac crest. Apply a slow, steady, medial force through the pelvic girdle. Maintain the force for 5 s. Positive test reproduces familiar pain in a symptomatic SIJ.

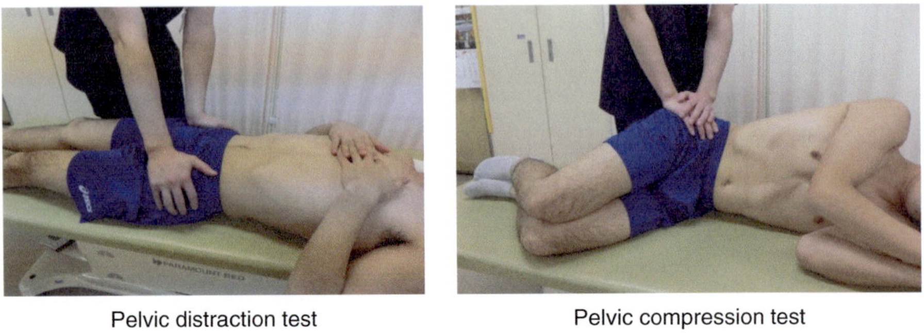

Fig. 4.6 Pelvic distraction test and pelvic compression test

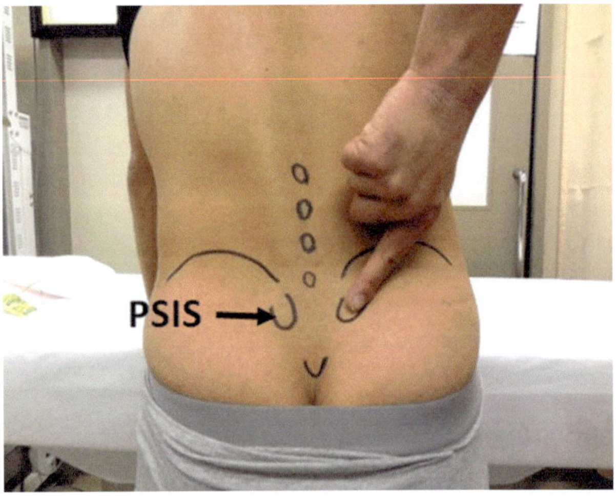

Fig. 4.7 The one-finger test

Morimoto et al. [6] indicate that positive rate of the sacroiliac joint shear test, Gaenslen's test, and Patrick's test in patients with SIJ disorder was 95%, 60%, and 45%, respectively.

4.2.2 The One-Finger Test (Fig. 4.7)

To accurately identify a pain area, we developed the one-finger test, where patients point to the main site of their pain using one finger [7].

We evaluated the relationship between pain area indicated by the one-finger test and effectiveness of SIJ injection (Fig. 4.8a). Eighteen of the 25 patients who indicated the main site of pain at or within 2 cm of the PSIS had an effective SIJ injection (Fig. 4.8b). And so, when a patient indicates within this circular area, there is a

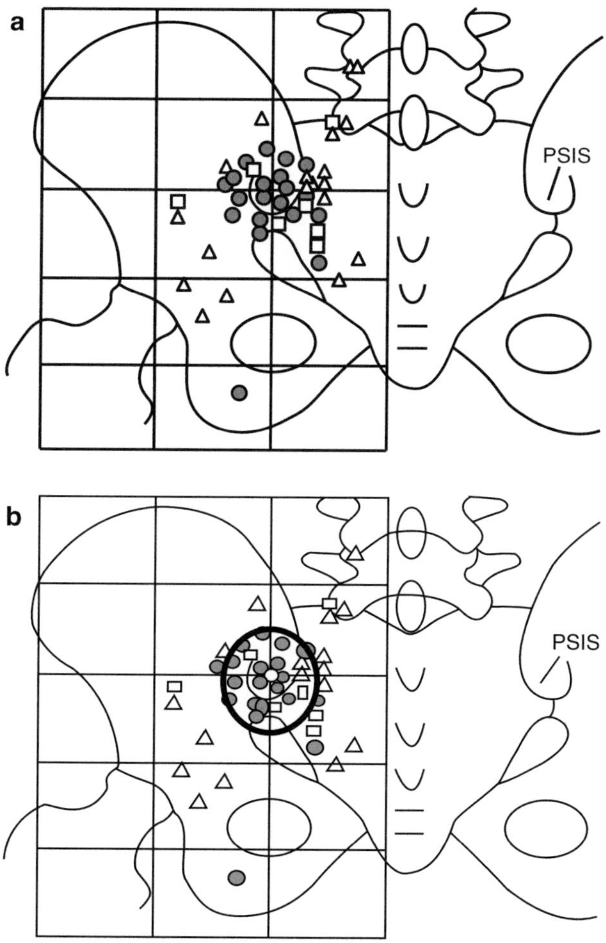

Fig. 4.8 Areas of pain indicated by patients with SIJ disorder. (**a**) The main sites of pain in 46 patients as indicated by the one-finger test. Square box: cases with a placebo response. Filled circle: cases with an effective SIJ injection. Triangle: cases with an ineffective SIJ injection. (**b**) When patients point to the area at or within 2cm of the PSIS (the area in a big circle) as the main site of pain by using one finger, the pain should be considered pain from the SIJ. With permission from [28]

high possibility they have SIJ disorder (Fig. 4.8b). This area is close to that indicated by the Fortin finger test [8].

In our recent data [9], 85% out of the patients with most painful area, indicated PSIS or around PSIS by the one-finger test, were diagnosed as those with SIJ pain (Fig. 4.9).

Key Message: The Difference Between the One-Finger Test and the Fortin Finger Test

The Fortin finger test is a test for indicating only SIJ disorder (Fig. 4.10a). On the other hand, the one-finger test is useful for detecting not only SIJ disorder but also other lesions such as facet joint pain, superior cluneal nerve entrapment, and sciatica (Fig. 4.10b).

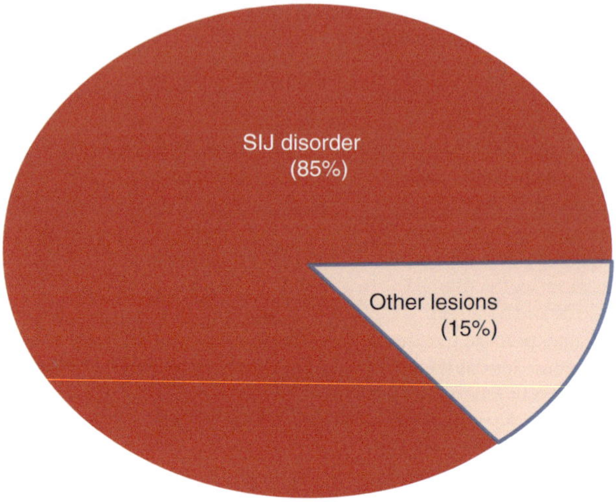

Fig. 4.9 Among patients with pain indicated at or around PSIS by the one-finger test, 85% of them was diagnosed as having SIJ disorder. With permission from [9]

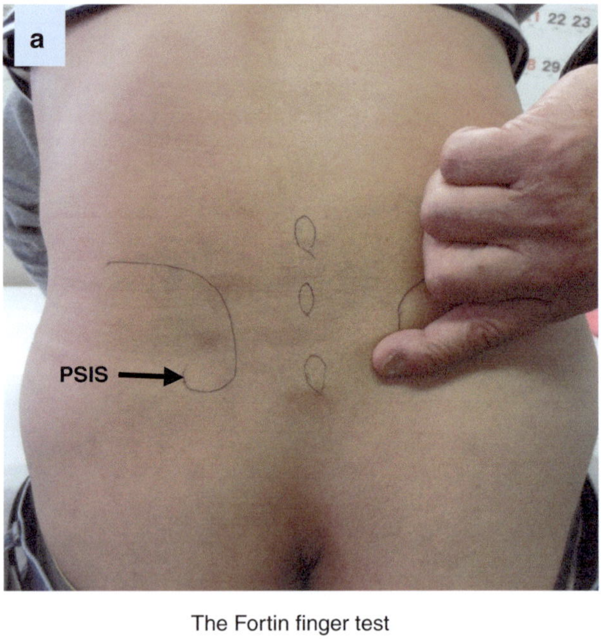

Fig. 4.10 (**a**) The Fortin finger test. Patients pointing to the area inferomedial to the PSIS within 1 cm with one finger should be those with SIJ disorder. (**b**) One-finger test is useful for detecting various lesions

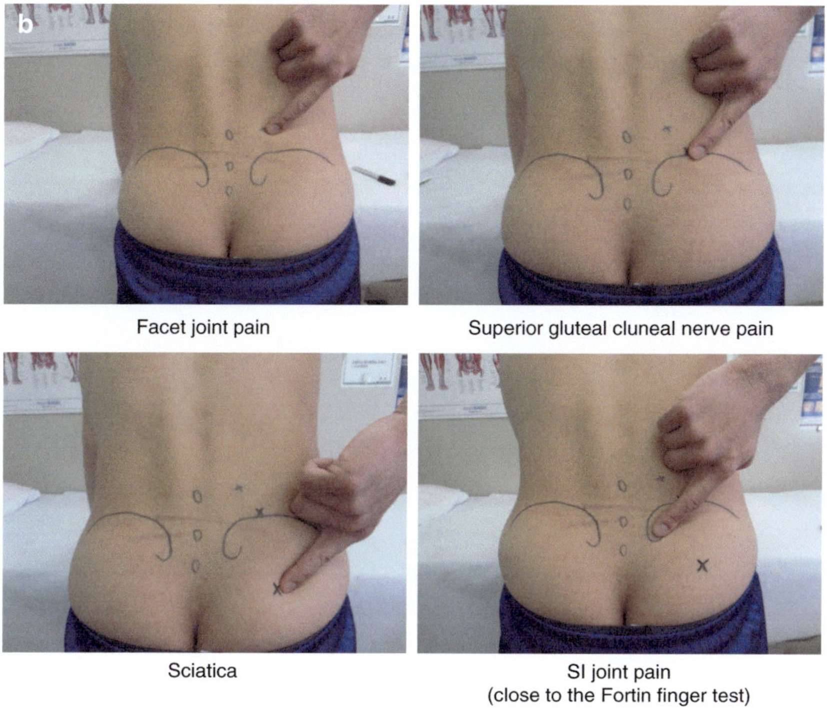

Fig. 4.10 (continued)

4.2.3 Tenderness Points Which Are Useful for Diagnosis

As mentioned earlier, tenderness points which are particularly useful for diagnosing SIJ pain include the PSIS, the long posterior sacroiliac ligament, the sacrotuberous ligament, and the iliac muscle [1].

Tips for palpating four tenderness points useful for diagnosing SIJ pain:

1. *PSIS: As the PSIS is a prominent area at the lower edge of the iliac crest, it can be touched, with the exception of obese patients (Fig. 4.11a).*
2. *Long posterior sacroiliac ligament: While you move your finger down from the PSIS, you should be able to touch the recessed ligamentous part and check the presence of tenderness there (Fig. 4.11b).*
3. *Sacrotuberous ligament: The patient lies prone with the lower limb internally rotated. If you have the patient relax the gluteal muscle, the ischial notch can be touched with your thumb. The sacrotuberous ligament can be palpated, as you slide your thumb cranially (Fig. 4.11c).*
4. *Iliac muscle: The patient lies supine with the patient' hip joint moderately flexed. You can touch the iliac muscles and check the presence or absence of tenderness in the iliac muscles while medially sliding a thumb deeply along the anterior superior iliac spine (ASIS) (Fig. 4.11d).*

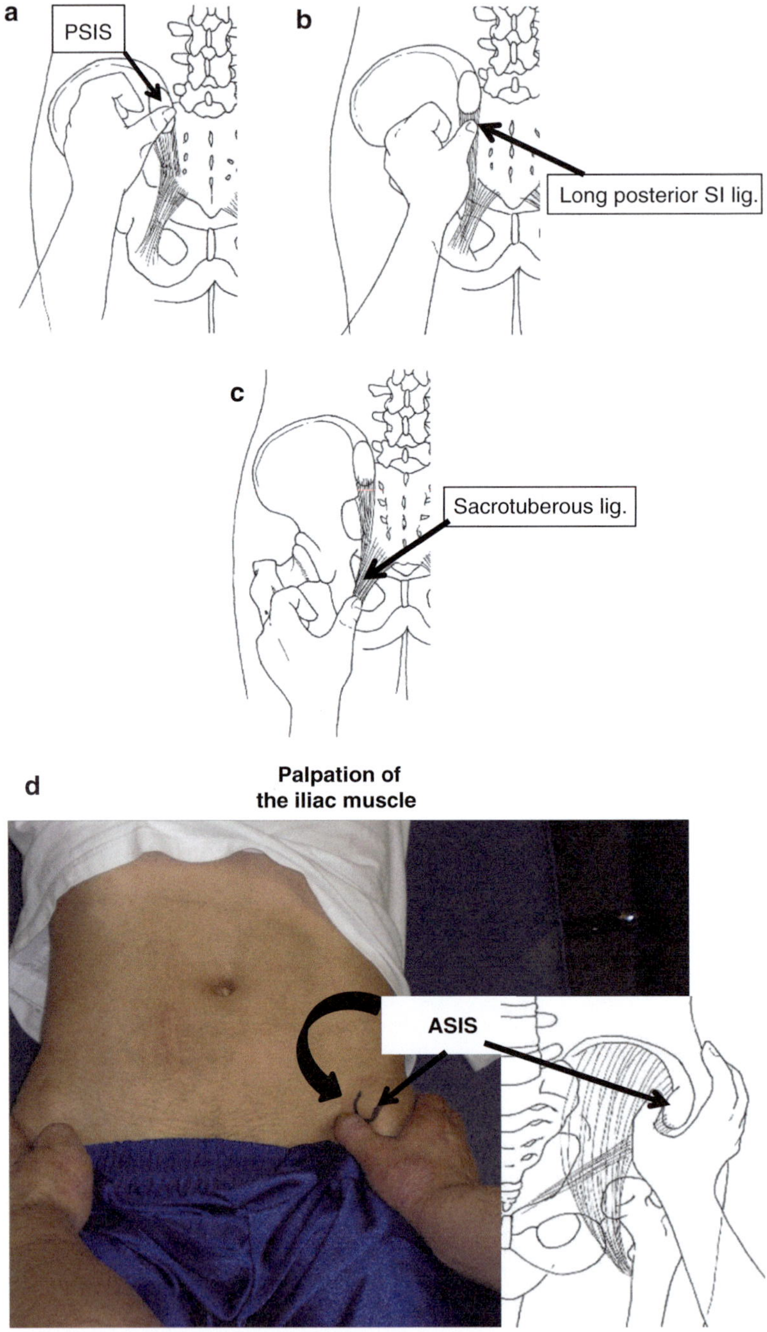

Fig. 4.11 (**a**) Tips for palpating the PSIS (**a**), the long posterior SI lig. (**b**), the sacrotuberous lig. (**c**), and the iliac muscle. (**d**) With permission from [28]

Key Message: Which Is Better to Identify the Pain Area, Using a Hand or One Finger?

When the area of low back pain is manually indicated by the patient using their hand, the outline of the pain area indicated was significantly wider than when indicated with only one finger [10] (Fig. 4.12). Moreover, it was also found that the pain area, which the patient complained of, was close to the area indicated using one finger. From this finding, we have determined that it is important to identify the extent of the pain area with one finger rather than with a hand.

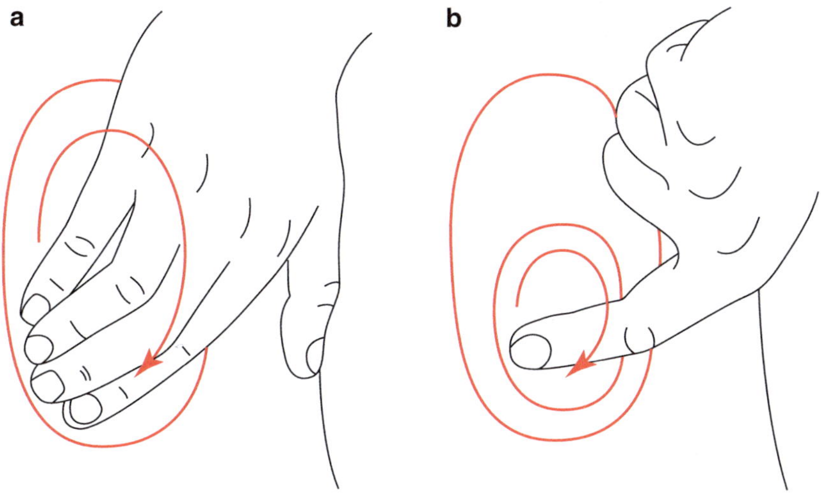

Fig. 4.12 Which is better to use a hand or a single finger to identify the pain area? (**a**) The outline of the pain area by using a hand. The indicated area was significantly wider than the actual pain area. (**b**) Identification using one finger is more localized and closer to the actual pain area. With permission from [28]

Table 4.1 Our inclusion criteria for SIJ disorder

1. Low back and/or buttock pain over the SIJ
2. Positive findings on at least one test among the sacroiliac shear test, Gaenslen's test, and Patrick's test
3. 70% or more pain relief after injection into the SIJ, after confirming injection into an another area, is ineffective

4.3 Diagnosis

4.3.1 The Criteria for Diagnosing SIJ Disorder

Cases which satisfy all of the conditions in Table 4.1 may be diagnosed as having typical SIJ disorder.

We often suspect SIJ disorder when conditions [1, 2] in Table 4.1 are positive, but we have thus far experienced some cases of SIJ disorder in which all the tests mentioned in [2] are negative. Therefore, even if condition [2] is not satisfied, when there is tenderness in the PSIS, long sacroiliac ligament, sacroiliac ligament, and iliac muscle, all of which are characteristic of SIJ disorder, it is worth trying an SIJ injection. Moreover, since according to our data [11], the one-finger test is positive in nearly 80% of cases of sacroiliac joint disorder, this test is useful for identifying the pain area. If the area near the PSIS is indicated by the one-finger test, there is a high possibility that the patient is suffering from SIJ disorder [9]. Finally, diagnosis of SIJ disorder is confirmed by SIJ injection with 70% or more pain relief.

4.3.2 Diagnostic Procedure for SIJ Disorder

Based on the understanding that SIJ dysfunction does not show abnormal findings directly linked to diagnosis on MRI or CT, the diagnosis of SIJ should be advanced. Rather, it should be considered that one of the features of the disease is low back pain without findings on images.

First, Pay Attention to the Gluteal Pain Area For the identification of the gluteal pain, the one-finger test mentioned above is useful. Second, pain provocation tests are performed. The sacroiliac joint shear test is especially effective for stress directly on the SIJ, while the Gaenslen's test and the Patrick's test are effective for stress through the femur. We usually use the sacroiliac joint shearing test because it has the highest positive rate among the three tests. In addition, if there is tenderness on any of the four points of the PSIS, long sacroiliac ligament, sacrotuberous ligament, and iliac muscle, it gives us additional useful information.

Ultimately, confirmed diagnosis is made by SIJ injection (Fig. 4.13).

4.3.3 Evaluation of Injection Effectiveness

The Effect Is Evaluated 15–30 Min After SIJ Injection However, there have been some cases in which the effectiveness of SIJ injection was not known until the next day. Moreover, there are other cases in which a combination of lumbar spinal lesions and SIJ disorder is present. Thus, the main ailment cannot be concretely determined only by the degree of symptom improvement or the duration of effectiveness of an SIJ injection.

Key Message: A Diagnostic Scoring System [1]
We developed a simple clinical diagnostic scoring system based on the accumulation of physical findings to distinguish between patients with SIJ pain and those with lumbar disc herniation or lumbar spinal stenosis. A scoring system based on multivariate logistic regression equations using the ten items investigated, characteristic of SIJ pain, was developed (Table 4.2).

Considering the positive rate and odds ratio, our scoring system consisted of only six items selected: the one-finger test (risk score 3 points), groin pain (risk score 2 points), and pain in sitting on a chair (risk score 1 point) and three physical examinations, the sacroiliac joint shear test, tenderness of PSIS, and sacrotuberous ligament (STL) (each, risk score 1 point) (Table 4.3).

The scoring system showed high sensitivity and specificity (a sensitivity of 90.3% and a specificity of 86.4% for a positivity cutoff point of 4, which is the sum of the scores) and is simple and easy to use in clinical practice. This scoring system is considered to help physicians and spine surgeons distinguish between patients with SIJ-related pain and those with lumbar disc herniation or lumbar spinal stenosis (Fig. 4.14).

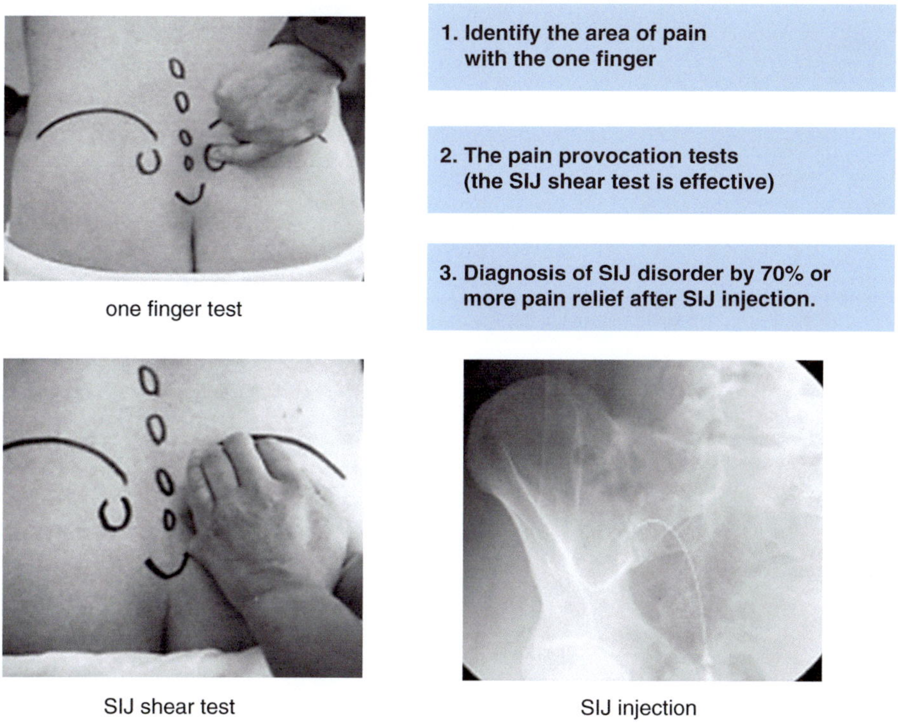

Fig. 4.13 Diagnostic procedure of SIJ disorder

Table 4.2 Investigating ten items

Pain area
1. One-finger test
Posterior superior iliac spine (PSIS) or not
2. Groin pain
Pain-increasing positions
3. Sitting on a chair without back rest
4. Supine
5. Lying on the painful side
Provocation test
6. Sacroiliac joint shear test (modified Newton's test)
Tenderness points
7. PSIS
8. Long posterior sacroiliac ligament (LPSL)
9. Sacrotuberous ligament (STL)
10. Iliac muscle

Table 4.3 A Diagnostic Scoring System

Items	Score
1. One-finger test	3
2. Groin pain	2
3. Sitting on the chair	1
4. Sacroiliac joint shear test	1
5. Tenderness of PSIS	1
6. Tenderness of STL	1
Total	9

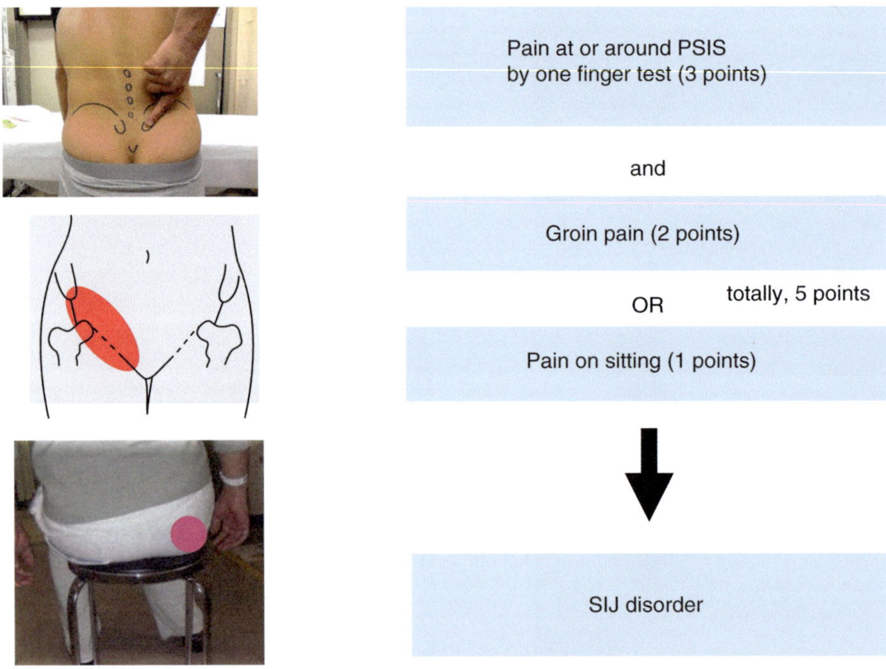

Fig. 4.14 To find SIJ disorder is not difficult

4.4 SIJ Injection

SIJ injection is the main method used for diagnosing SIJ disorder.

4.4.1 Two Types of SIJ Injection (Intra-articular and Peri-articular) (Fig. 4.15)

It is known that there are two types of SIJ injection, intra-articular and peri-articular SIJ injection.

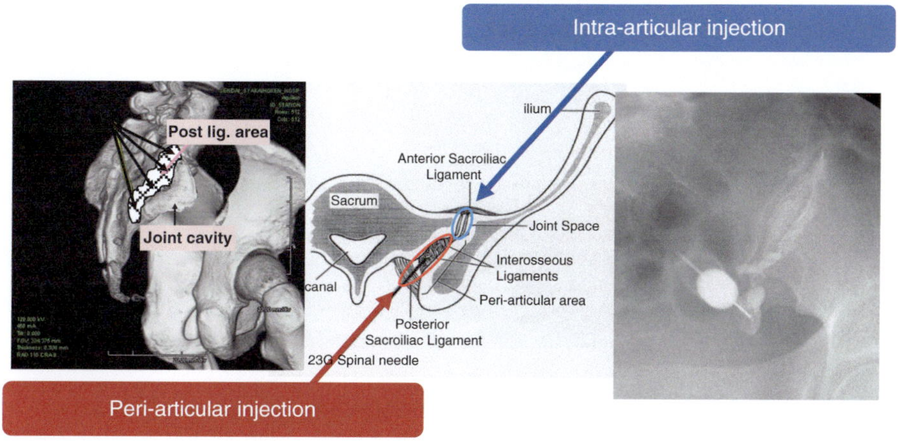

Fig. 4.15 Two types of SIJ injections. There are two types of SIJ injections: intra-articular and peri-articular. An intra-articular SIJ injection is injected into the articular compartment, and a peri-articular SIJ injection is injected into the posterior ligamentous compartment

For an intra-articular SIJ injection, the needle is inserted into the articular compartment. For a peri-articular SIJ injection, the needle is inserted into the ligamentous compartment.

4.4.2 Intra-articular Injection (Fig. 4.16a)

4.4.2.1 The Diagnostic Rate by Intra-articular Injection Is Low

Until now, it has been thought that intra-articular injections could be the gold standard for diagnosing patients with SIJ disorder. However, the diagnostic rates of patients with SIJ pain using intra-articular injection in previous studies [12–15] were not high, ranging from 18 to 60%.

4.4.2.2 The Reason for the Low Diagnostic Rate by Intra-articular Injection

Borowsky et al. [16] reported that performing both intra-articular injection and peri-articular injection was more effective than only intra-articular injection for SIJ disorder. Thus, the posterior ligaments (peri-articular region) should also be a target of diagnostic injections because only performing intra-articular injections could contribute to an underestimation in the prevalence of SIJ pain. Recent European guidelines do not also recommend diagnosing SIJ disorder using only an intra-articular injection. Dall et al. [17] wrote in their book that if the intra-articular injection was negative, an extra-articular injection should be considered.

In our study [18], we concluded that pain from SIJ disorder originates from both the intra- and peri-articular region, but the peri-articular region might be more often responsible, because a peri-articular injection was more effective than an intra-articular injection for SIJ disorder (improvement rate, 96% vs 62%).

Fig. 4.16 Intra-articular SIJ injection

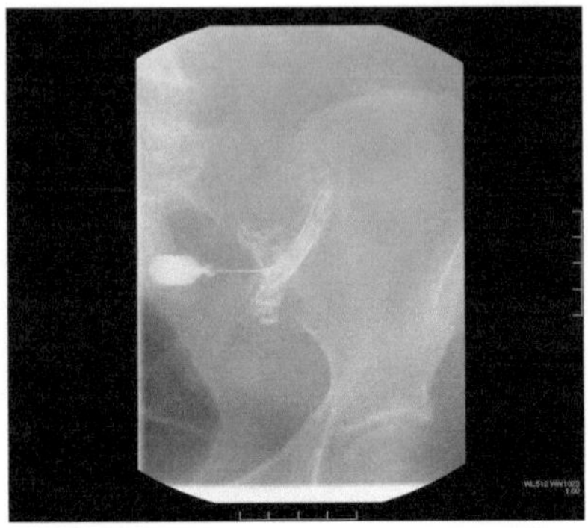

4.4.2.3 Intra-articular Injections Are Technically Not Easy to Perform

The success rate of the intra-articular injection was reported as 20% [16] and 80% [12]. As Maigne [12] is an SIJ specialist, his rate is not the norm. We can assume that this injection is difficult to perform for general physicians who are not familiar with the SIJ.

The injection method developed by Hendrix et al. [19] is considered to be the conventional method for an intra-articular injection used worldwide. However, many physicians using the method should understand it is not actually easy to perform. The main reason for this is that the injection needle is not always inserted into the joint cavity, even if the joint space is visible. As the joint cavity is occupied by joint cartilage, the joint space visible under fluoroscopic imaging may not be the actual cavity (Dhilmann W: Diagnostic Radiology of the Sacroiliac Joints. Georg Thieme Verlag, Stuttgart, New York, 1980, pp. 1–2). Until now, the difficulty of the intra-articular injection has made diagnosis and treatment of the disease difficult.

4.4.3 Peri-articular Injection (Fig. 4.17)

4.4.3.1 A Peri-articular Injection Is Much Easier to Perform than an Intra-articular Injection

We developed a method for peri-articular injections [18]. The posterior ligamentous region of the SIJ is divided into four equal sections. An injection needle is inserted roughly into the center of each area. Local anesthetics is injected only into areas in which familiar pain can be reproduced by needle irritation. We can usually perform this injection successfully under fluoroscopic guidance. Any physician, even a resident, should be able to perform this injection successfully.

4.4.3.2 Most SIJ Disorders Can Be Diagnosed by Using a Peri-articular Injection

Our recent data [9] showed that about 80% of patients with SIJ disorder had pain relief by a peri-articular injection, and merely about 20% of the patients required an

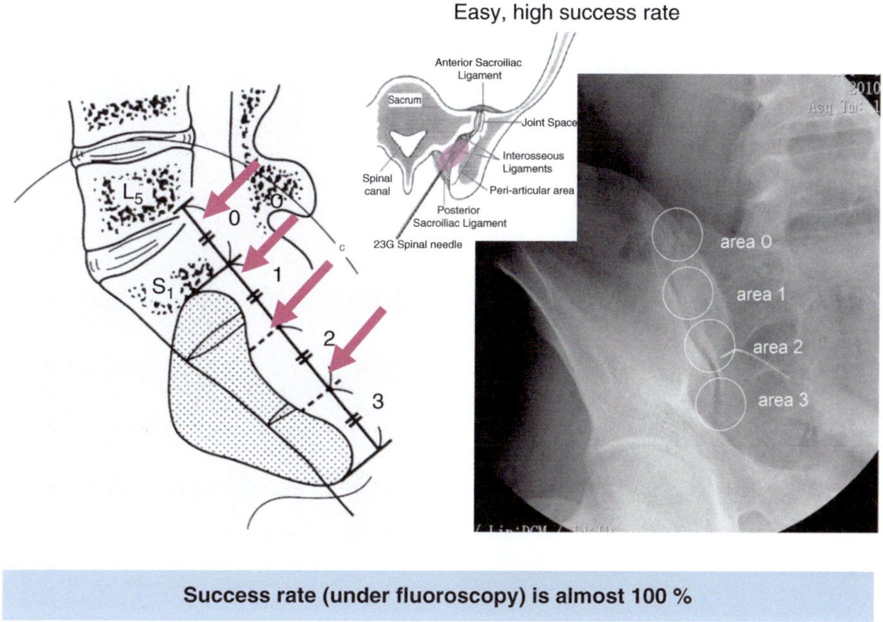

Fig. 4.17 Peri-articular injection

Fig. 4.18 Peri-articular SIJ injection was effective in 81% of patients with gluteal pain around the PSIS as indicated by the one-finger test [9]

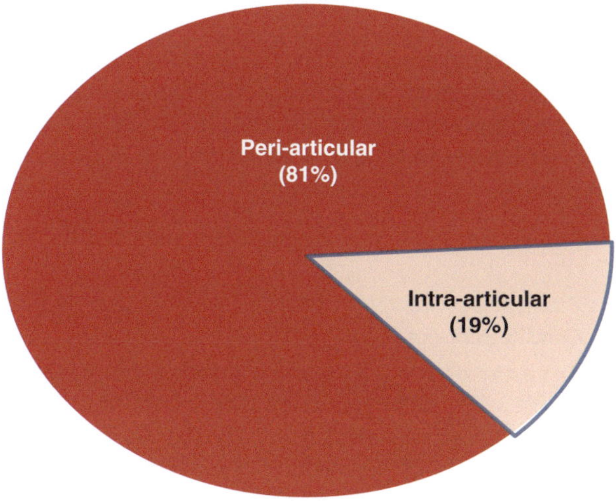

additional intra-articular injection (Fig. 4.18). This means that the origin of most SIJ disorder is situated in the peri-articular region, such as the posterior ligamentous region. That is to say, most SIJ disorder can be diagnosed by a peri-articular injection.

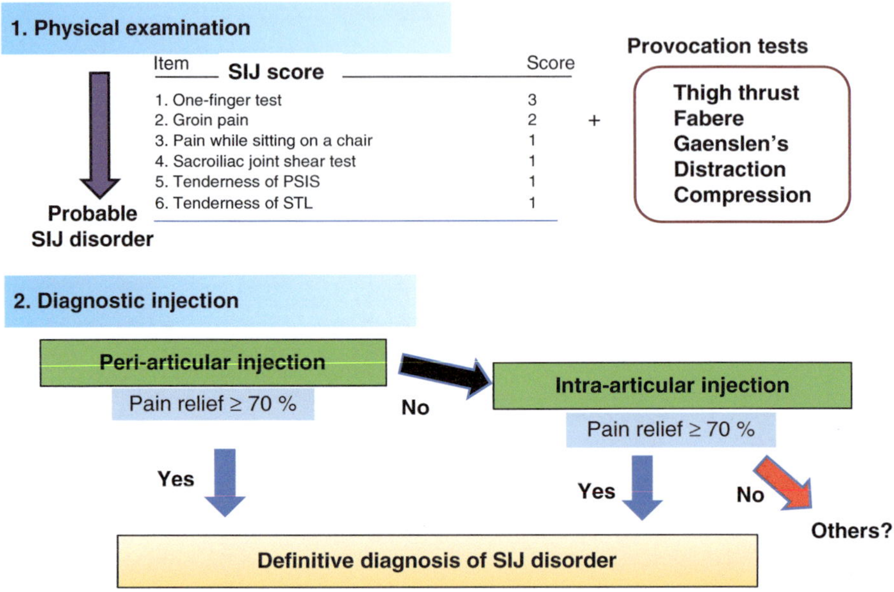

Fig. 4.19 Diagnostic algorithm for SIJ disorder in Japan

4.4.4 A Diagnostic Algorithm for SIJ Disorder

We recommend the following diagnostic algorithm for SIJ disorder as it is generally performed in Japan: while suspecting SIJ disorder based on the results of physical examinations, such as provocation tests and SIJ scores, first a peri-articular injection should be performed, and, if ineffective, an intra-articular injection should be done (Fig. 4.19).

Key Message: Our Theory for Two Types of Injection Corresponding to the Condition of the SIJ (Fig. 4.20)

Two types of injection may be required corresponding to the condition of the SIJ.

A peri-articular injection may be suitable for pain originating from the posterior ligamentous region, such as SIJ dysfunction, and an intra-articular injection may be required for arthritis and synovitis in the cavity.

The most pathological condition in the SIJ is thought to be dysfunction. It is supposed that in a small amount of patients suffering from prolonged dysfunction, arthritis can develop in the cavity, as well as (in addition to) synovitis from seronegative spondyloarthropathy.

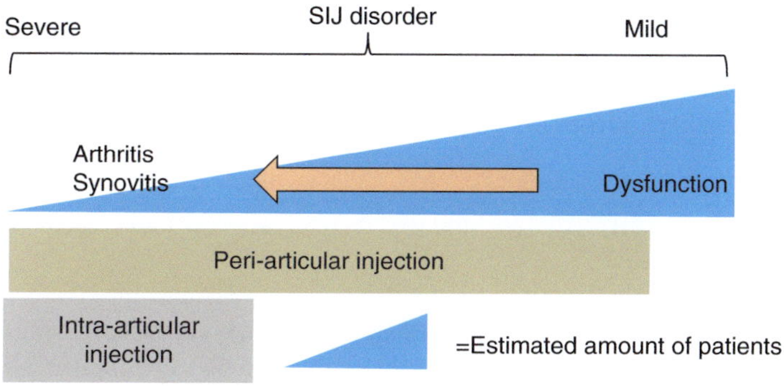

Fig. 4.20 Arthritis in the cavity can develop in a small number of patients suffering from prolonged dysfunction

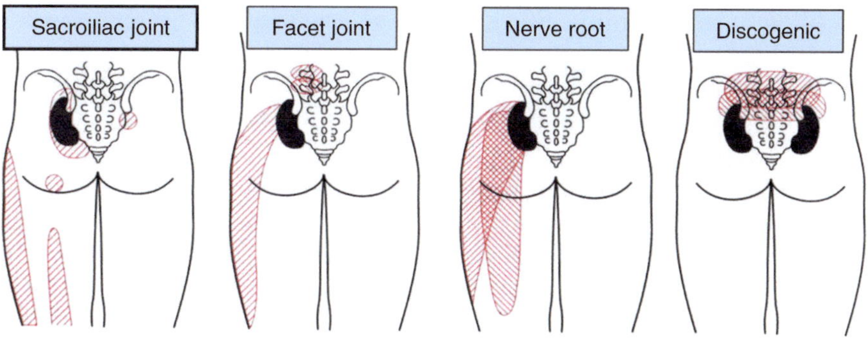

Fig. 4.21 Differentiation of SIJ disorder from lumbar spine diseases by judging the pain area. With permission from [28]

4.5 Differential Diagnosis

4.5.1 Differentiation Between SIJ Disorder and Lumbar Spinal Diseases

4.5.1.1 Degenerative Lumbar Spine Diseases Differentiated by Pain Area (Fig. 4.21) [20]

Pain from the lumbar facet joint involves referred pain that spreads into the thigh. In some patients pain extends to the SIJ region. However, the focus of the referred pain is not on the SIJ, so it can be distinguished from pain related to the SIJ.

Even pain from injured nerve roots may be applied to the SIJ area, but the focus of the pain is close to the center of the buttocks, not the SIJ, so it can be distinguished from SIJ pain. However, we have experienced cases where pain from an injured S1 nerve root is confined near the PSIS. So, caution is required as there are some cases which are difficult to distinguish from SIJ disorder.

Pain derived from intervertebral discs has an unclear border and often extends from one side of the body, beyond the spinous process and into the opposite side. However, because pain derived from intervertebral discs is not focused on the SIJ, it can be distinguished from SIJ pain.

Key Message: Tips for Distinguishing Between SIJ Disorder and Degenerative Lumbar Spine Diseases

When distinguishing between pain from SIJ disorder and that from lumbar spine disease, it is important to know where the pain is focused most intensely. The one-finger test is useful in finding the focus of pain. In addition, confirming whether or not pain is induced by the SIJ shear test, which puts a direct load on the SIJ, can help us distinguish between SIJ disorder and lumbar spine disease.

Most patients with SIJ disorder feel the most intense pain around the PSIS. In contrast, for patients with lumbar spine disease, the focus of pain is rarely near the PSIS, and pain is not induced by SIJ shear test as well.

4.5.1.2 Spinal Metastasis Caused by Cancer

With this condition, a history of malignant tumors and abnormal findings from the vertebral body to the pedicle on an MRI are recognized. Low back pain occurs when the vertebral body causes a compressed fracture. Paying attention to the pain site and the result of the SIJ sear test makes differentiation between pain from spinal metastasis and pain from SIJ disorder possible, because the test does not usually induce pain in this condition.

4.5.1.3 Pyogenic Spondylitis

In this condition, heavy low back pain accompanied by fever and an increase of CRP and WBC in blood tests are observed. A high signal in the intervertebral discs and epidural abscesses are sometimes seen on an MRI. The SIJ sear test is not likely to induce pain near the PSIS, and pain from the disease is usually localized at the low back region.

4.5.1.4 Osteoporotic Vertebral Compression Fracture

An MRI examination is useful and indispensable for determining whether the compression fracture is a fresh fracture or not. Pain originating from a compression fracture manifests itself as back pain around the fracture site. However, it is important to bear in mind that some patients who have this condition complain of having SIJ disorder. It is thought that as thoracic kyphosis caused by a compression fracture progresses, SIJ pain develops, owing to an increased load on the SIJ.

4.5.2 Noteworthy Pain Which Originates from Around the SIJ (Fig. 4.22a)

In order to identify pain from these diseases as follows, the one-finger test should be effective (Fig. 4.22b).

4.5.2.1 Entrapment Neuropathy of the Superior Cluneal Nerve [21]

Most patients with entrapment neuropathy of the superior cluneal nerve have tenderness on the iliac crest 7–8 cm laterally from the spinous process of the lumbar spine where the nerve passes along. As well, the one-finger test indicates a point of tenderness over the iliac crest. Hence, finding the disease should not be difficult. Patients with entrapment neuropathy often have pain spreading into the gluteal region and sometimes the lower leg. Pain develops when standing from a sitting position, when rotating, or by bending the lumbar spine laterally.

4.5.2.2 Iliolumbar Ligament Syndrome [22]

The iliolumbar ligament originates from the L5 transverse process and attaches to the iliac crest. When the human body transitions from a bent forward standing position to an erect position, the iliolumbar ligament bears the most load. Thus, the syndrome is likely to develop in daily life. The syndrome is easily diagnosed by finding tenderness near the tip of the L5 transverse process. Injecting a local anesthetic into the point of tenderness should be effective.

4.5.2.3 Sacrotuberous Ligament Syndrome [23]

The sacrotuberous ligament attaches to the lower part of the sacrum and the sciatic tuberosity (or the ligament connects A to B). It is characteristic that most patients with this syndrome have tenderness on the lower part of the sacrum and the sciatic tuberosity. Injecting a local anesthetic into the point of tenderness of the ligament should be effective.

4.5.2.4 Piriformis Syndrome [24]

Piriformis syndrome is characterized as causing the sciatica by continuous contraction of the piriformis muscle which compresses the sciatic nerve. With this syndrome, tenderness is characteristically present on the piriformis muscle or on an entrapment site of the nerve. An injection of a local anesthetic for diagnosis and treatment of the syndrome is given.

4.5.2.5 Entrapment Neuropathy of the Superior Gluteal Nerve [25]

The superior gluteal nerve often becomes entrapped in the superior foramen of the piriformis muscle. With this syndrome, tenderness is characteristically present on an entrapment site of the nerve. The release around the superior gluteal nerve by injecting physiologic saline should also be effective.

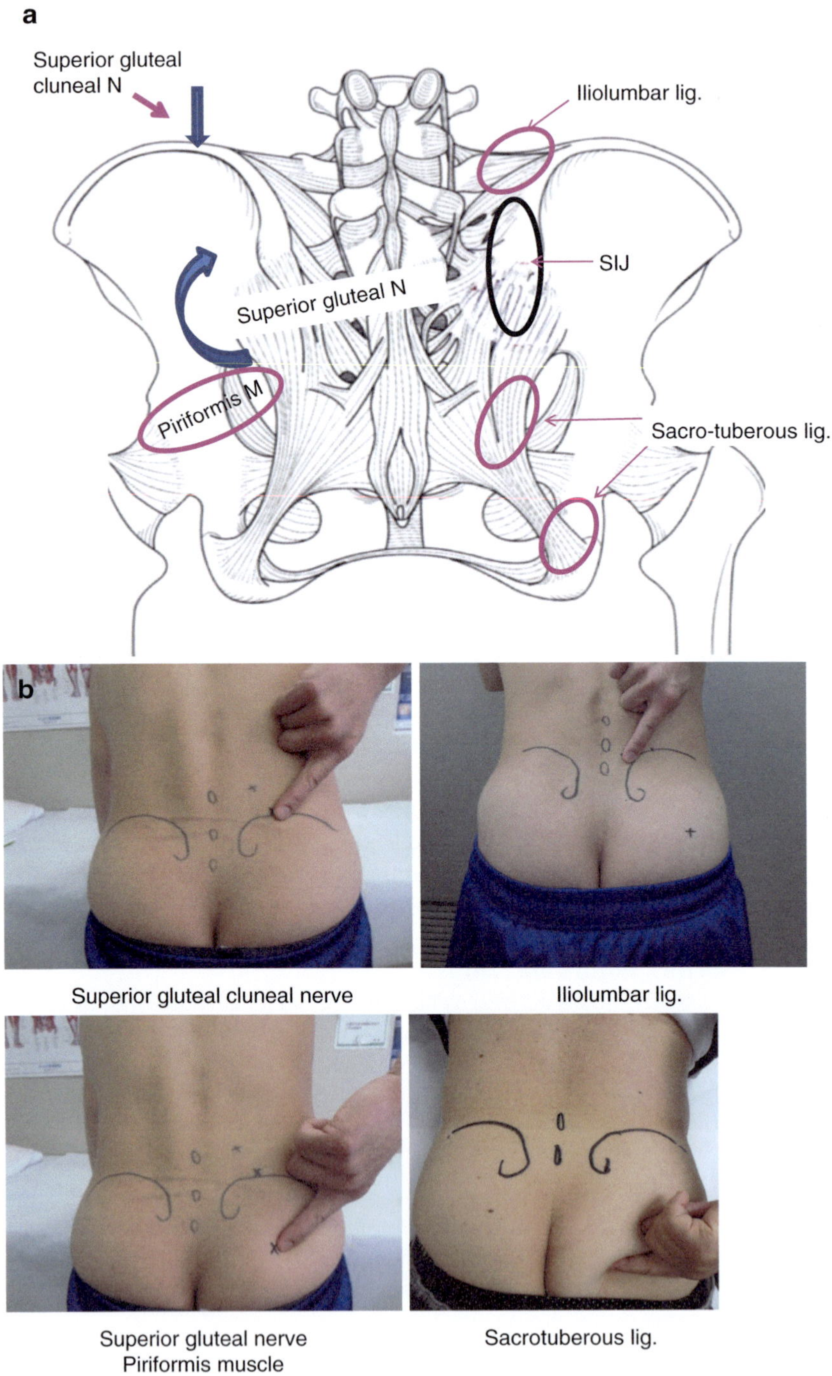

Fig. 4.22 (**a**) Pain originating from around the SIJ. (**b**) The one-finger test should be effective for detecting pain from diseases around the SIJ

After the release of the nerve, patients could stand and walk more stably as well as feel pain relief. These injections can be successfully performed by confirming the muscle or the superior gluteal artery around the nerve using an ultrasound device.

4.5.3 Relationship Between the Hip Joint and SIJ

As recognized in hip-spine syndrome, there is a generally accepted close relationship between the hip joint and the lumbar spine. However, the SIJ is located closer to the hip joint than the lumbar spine. As both joints cause groin pain, the pain from both joints are easily misunderstood.

In order to differentiate groin pain originating from the hip joint and that originating from the SIJ, it is first necessary to confirm whether the space of the hip joint is narrow in an X-ray image. However, there are some patients with groin pain relieved by SIJ injection; nevertheless their X-rays show findings of hip joint arthrosis. Therefore, careful examination is necessary in order to distinguish the two. It is important to confirm whether pain is induced by the SIJ shear test, which puts a direct load on the SIJ.

Key Message: Sports Injuries Which Are Caused by SIJ Disorder
Recently, attention is paid to athletes who suffer from groin pain. Repair of the covering tissues around the groin region has been performed on many athletes. However, a recent report has stated that sports injuries in young people often relate to the SIJ [26]. It is necessary to differentiate a groin tissue injury from groin pain caused by SIJ disorders, because groin pain is characteristic of SIJ disorders. *We should bear in mind that groin pain accompanied by low back pain is often caused by SIJ disorder* [1].

Key Message: Pain at the Posterior Area of the Greater Trochanter Which Cannot Be Relieved by an SIJ Injection
SIJ disorder sometimes induces pain at the posterior area of the greater trochanter which is not easily relieved by SIJ injection.

In many cases, patients have tenderness corresponding to the area where the piriform muscle is attached to the greater trochanter of the femur. An injection of local anesthetic and a steroid into the area is effective because the pain is most likely being induced by an inflammation in the area.

4.5.4 Organ Diseases Which Should Be Differentiated from SIJ Disorder [27]

There are some organ diseases that show pain which can be confused with that of SIJ disorder.

However, a change in posture does not commonly increase pain from organ diseases. Moreover, a pain provocation test, such as the SIJ shear test, is useful in differentiating organ diseases from SIJ disorder because the test adds direct stress on the SIJ. This is less likely to produce a positive result in organ diseases.

4.5.4.1 Obstetrics and Gynecological Diseases

An MRI examination is effective for diagnosis.

Endometriosis

Low back pain is frequently observed and accompanied by dysmenorrhea, lower abdominal pain, and pain during sexual intercourse.

In addition, ectopic endometriosis, which occurs near the sciatic nerve or the sacral plexus, stimulates the nerves in conjunction with (during) the menstrual cycle, and so lower limb pain (periodic sciatica) develops. In some cases, the piriformis muscle is compressed by the disease and causes the piriformis syndrome.

Ovarian Cyst, Ovarian Cancer

Some cases can cause pain from the low back to the pelvic region.

Uterine Myoma, Uterine Retroflexion

Some cases can cause low back pain.

4.5.4.2 Urological Diseases

Urinary Tract Stone

A characteristic of which is intermittent episode of paroxysmal low back pain on one side. For diagnosis, a confirmation by X-ray image and a urine examination for hematuria are necessary.

Pyelonephritis

Complications for which include fever, nausea, and dull low back pain. A urine examination shows increased white blood cells and bacteria in urine. Intense (severe) pain can be observed in the costovertebral angle (CVA) on one side.

Kidney Cancer

When it has progressed, low back pain on one side develops. MRI is useful for diagnosis.

4.5.4.3 Lung Cancer

Lung cancer with spinal metastasis causes low back pain, as well as chest pain and cough.

4.5.4.4 Digestive Diseases

Stomach/duodenal ulcers, stomach cancer, acute/chronic pancreatitis, pancreatic cancer, and gallstones/cholecystitis also cause back pain. The patient's past history and amylase value should be checked. MRI and CT are useful for diagnosis.

4.5.4.5 Disorders of the Blood System

Multiple Myeloma

This is often treated as osteoporosis. In this condition, blood sedimentation is often high.

The presence of Bence-Jones protein is helpful for diagnosis.

Spinal Metastasis of Malignant Lymphoma

Findings via MRI and a blood examination are useful for diagnosis.

4.5.4.6 Vascular Diseases

A dissecting abdominal aortic aneurysm is accompanied by an intense low back pain and is often followed by a state of shock. The onset time should be clear and a delay in diagnosis can cause fatal results. It is always important and necessary to distinguish this disease from common low back pain. An enhanced CT examination is essential for a more detailed confirmation.

4.5.4.7 Psychogenic Low Back Pain

There are patients whose psychiatric problems are the main cause of low back pain.

Patients with somatoform disorders, such as somatization disorders, convertible disorders, hypochondriasis, pain disorders, etc., and psychosomatic diseases sometimes complain of chronic low back pain.

References

1. Kurosawa D, Murakami E, Ozawa H, et al. A diagnostic scoring system for sacroiliac joint pain originating from the posterior ligament. Pain Med. 2017;18:228–38.
2. Dreyfuss P, Michaelsen M, Pausa K, et al. The value of medical history and physical examination in diagnosing sacroiliac joint pain. Spine. 1996;21:2594–602.
3. Berthelot JM, Labat JJ, Le Goff B, Gouin F, Maugars Y. Provocative sacroiliac joint maneuvers and sacroiliac joint block are unreliable for diagnosing sacroiliac joint pain. Joint Bone Spine. 2006;73:17–23.
4. Kim YH, Yao Z, Kim K, Park WM. Quantitative investigation of ligament strains during physical tests for sacroiliac joint pain using finite element analysis. Man Ther. 2014;19:235–41.
5. Laslett M, Aprill CN, Mcdonald B, Young SB. Diagnosis of sacroiliac joint pain: validity of individual provocation tests and composites of tests. Man Ther. 2005;10:207–2018.
6. Morimoto D, Isu T, Kim K, et al. Treatment of sacroiliac joint dysfunction. Spinal Surg. 2010;24:6–11. (in Japanese).
7. Murakami E, Aizawa T, Kanno H, et al. Diagram specific to the sacroiliac joint pain indicated by one-finger test. J Orthop Sci. 2008;13:492–7.
8. Fortin JD, Falco FJE. The Fortin finger test: an indicator of sacroiliac pain. Am J Orthop. 1997;26:477–80.

9. Murakami E, Kurosawa D, Aizawa T. Treatment strategy for sacroiliac joint-related pain at or around the posterior superior iliac spine. Clin Neurol Neurosurg. 2018;165:43–6.
10. Kanno H, Murakami E. Comparison of low back pain sites identified by patient's finger versus hand: prospective randomized controlled clinical trial. J Orthop Sci. 2007;12:254–9.
11. Tanaka H, Murakami E, Kurosawa D, et al. A study for features of lumbar lesions including sacroiliac joint disorder by the one finger test. J Jpn Orthop Assoc. 2011;85:S589. (in Japanese).
12. Maigne JY, Aivalikis A, Pfefer F. Results of sacroiliac joint double block and value of sacroiliac pain provocation tests in 54 patients with low back pain. Spine. 1996;2:1889–92.
13. Schwarzer AC, Aprill CN, Bogduk N. The sacroiliac joint in chronic low back pain. Spine. 1995;20:31–7.
14. Young S, April C, Laslett M. Correlation of clinical examination characteristics with three sources of chronic low back pain. Spine J. 2003;3:460–5.
15. Slipman CW, Sterenfeld EB, Chou LH, et al. The predictive value of provocative sacroiliac joint stress maneuvers in the diagnosis of sacroiliac syndrome. Arch Phys Med Rehabil. 1998;79:288–92.
16. Borowsky CD, Fagen G. Sources of sacroiliac region pain: insights gained from a study comparing standard intra-articular injection with a technique combining intra-and periarticular injection. Arch Phys Med Rehabil. 2008;89:2048–56.
17. Dall BE, Eden SV, Rahl MD, Smith AG. Algorithm for the diagnosis and treatment of the dysfunctional sacroiliac joint. In: Dall BE, editor. Surgery for the painful, dysfunctional sacroiliac joint. Cham: Springer; 2014. p. 62.
18. Murakami E, Tanaka Y, Aizawa T, et al. Effect of peri-articular and intra-articular injections for sacroiliac joint pain: a prospective comparative study. J Orthop Sci. 2007;12:274–80.
19. Hendrix RW, Lin PP, Kane WJ. Simplified aspiration of injection technique for the sacroiliac joint. J Bone Joint Surg Am. 1982;64:1249–52.
20. Murakami E, Ishizuka M, Kokubun S, et al. Clinical features of motion-related sacroiliac joint pain. Clin Orthop Surg. 1997;32:387–92. (in Japanese).
21. Morimoto D, Isu T, Kim K, et al. Surgical treatment of superior cluneal nerve entrapment neuropathy. J Neurosurg Spine. 2013;19:71–5.
22. Naeim F, Froetscher L, Hirshberg GG. Treatment of the chronic iliolumbar syndrome by infiltration of the iliolumbar ligament. West J Med. 1982;136:372–4.
23. Hackett GS. Referred pain from low back ligament disability. AMA Arch Surg. 1956;73:878–83.
24. Robinson DR. Piriformis syndrome in relation to sciatic pain. Am J Surg. 1947;73:355–8.
25. Rask MR. Superior gluteal nerve entrapment syndrome. Muscle Nerve. 1980;3:304–7.
26. Prather H. Sacroiliac joint pain: practical management. Clin J Sport Med. 2003;13:252–5.
27. Yoshimoto M. In: Nakamura K, Yamashita T, editors. Youtsu. Clinical practice (in Japanese). Tokyo: Nakayama-Syoten; 2010. p. 248–54.
28. Murakami E. Sacroiliac joint pain: undiagnosed low back pain. Tokyo: Nankodo; 2012. (in Japanese).

Treatment of Sacroiliac Joint Disorder

5

Abstract

- Most cases are treated by conservative therapies using an SIJ injection, drugs, or a manual therapy.
- SIJ injection is the first choice for the treatment of SIJ disorder.
- Peri-articular injection can be more effective in most patients with SIJ disorder than intra-articular injection.
- The algorithm that first, a peri-articular injection, and if ineffective, an intra-articular injection should be performed will allow us easily to treat more patients with SIJ disorder.
- Recent methods of SIJ fusion, such as iFuse Implant System, DIANA, and our anterior approach should be thought as being beneficial in pain relief but used only as a final means of treatment for SIJ disorder.

5.1 Treatment Strategy for SIJ Disorder

Most cases are treated by conservative treatments. For cases in which the effect of the injection does not last even while making full use of conservative therapy, the fusion of the SIJ should be considered as the final means to rescue.

5.2 Conservative Treatments

5.2.1 SIJ Injection

SIJ injection is the first choice for the treatment of SIJ disorder.

E. Murakami, *Sacroiliac Joint Disorder*,
https://doi.org/10.1007/978-981-13-1807-8_5

5.2.1.1 The Origin of Most SIJ Disorder Is Probably Located in the Peri-articular Region

As mentioned in Chap. 4, there are two types of SIJ injection: the intra-articular and the peri-articular injection (Fig. 5.1). However, for most physicians, the intra-articular injection is technically not as easy as the peri-articular injection to perform. In our previous study [1], a peri-articular injection was more effective than an intra-articular injection for SIJ disorder. This indicates that the origin of most SIJ disorder is probably located in the peri-articular region, such as the posterior ligamentous region. Our findings are supported by previous studies [2, 3]. Lee et al. [2] reported that botulinum toxin injected into the posterior SI ligaments showed clinical usefulness in pain reduction and for functional improvement in patients with SIJ pain. Furthermore, Fukui et al. [3] showed the effectiveness of pulsed radiofrequency applied to the sacroiliac ligaments for SIJ pain. Thus, a peri-articular injection would be the most direct approach into the origin of most SIJ disorder.

Our recent data [4] shows that a peri-articular injection was effective in about 80% of patients with typical SIJ disorder, and only the remaining 20% of patients required an additional intra-articular injection. This shows that in most patients, the peri-articular injection is effective for diagnosis and treatment of SIJ disorder.

We recommend the following strategy to treat SIJ disorder (Fig. 5.2):

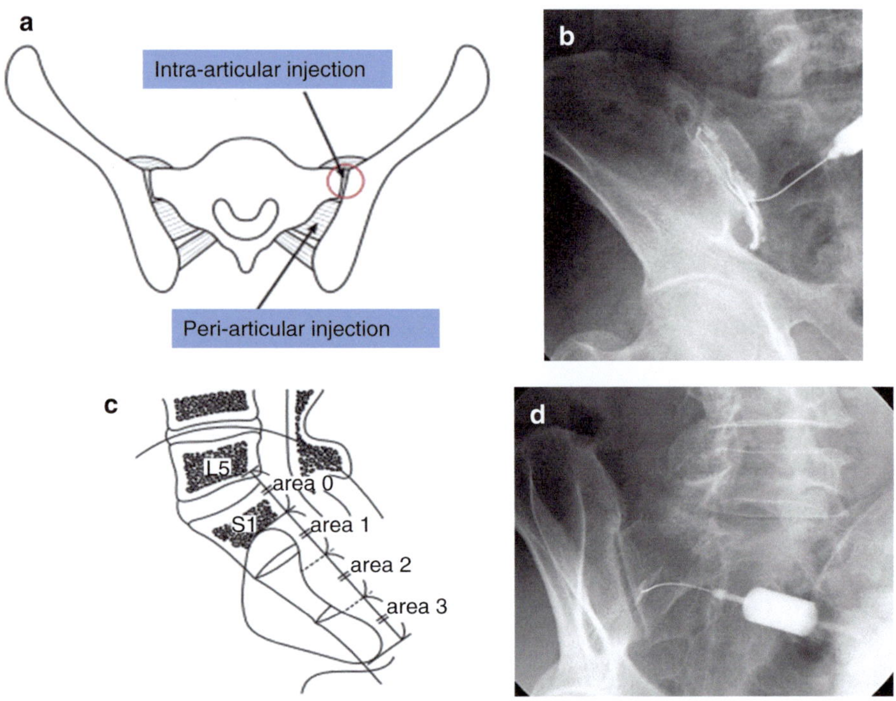

Fig. 5.1 SIJ injections. (**a**) Two types of SIJ injections: intra-articular injection into the articular compartment and peri-articular injection into the posterior ligamentous compartment. (**b**) Arthrogram of the joint cavity. (**c**) The four divided sections (area 0 ~ 3) of the posterior peri-articular area of SIJ. (**d**) Arthrogram in Area 2 of the SIJ

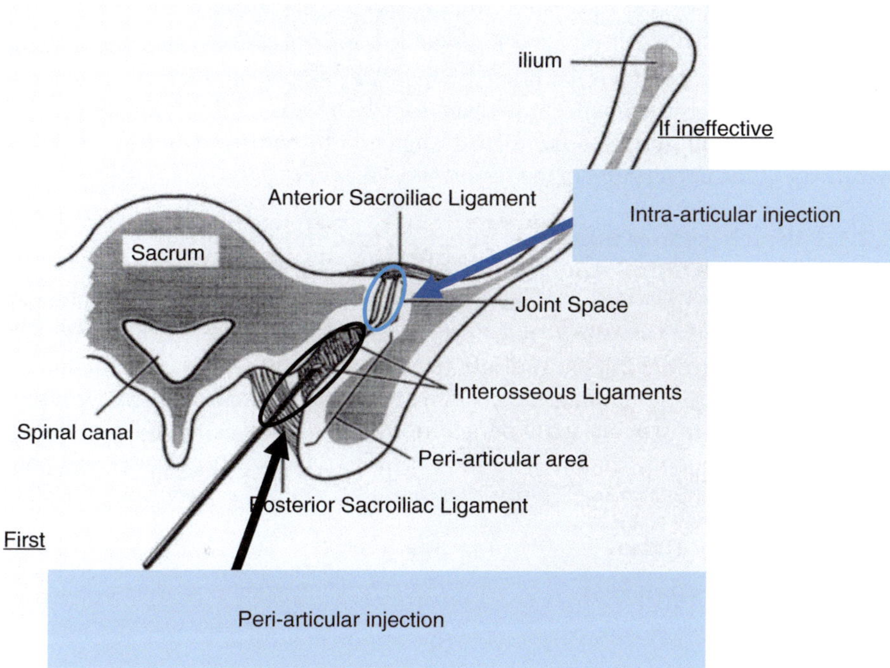

Fig. 5.2 Strategy for treating SIJ disorder

Fig. 5.3 A probable mechanism of pain relief by an injection

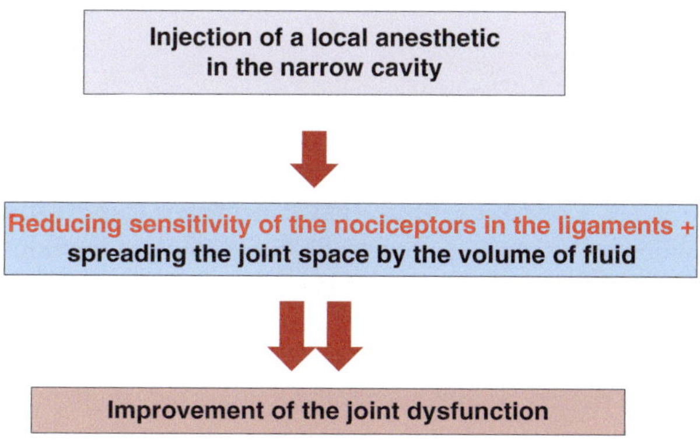

A peri-articular injection should be performed first, and if the peri-articular injection is ineffective, an intra-articular injection should be added. Using this algorithm, more cases of SIJ disorder can be easily treated.

5.2.1.2 Mechanism of Pain Relief by an Injection (Fig. 5.3)

How Can an Injection of Local Anesthetic Relieve Pain for a Long Period of Time?
The lasting effect of an injected local anesthetic (lidocaine) is at most 2–3 h. However, in the SIJ, it often lasts for a few days and in some cases several weeks.

The effect beyond the pharmacological limit of the local anesthetic drug cannot be explained only in terms of the pharmacological effect. Based on this fact, the following mechanism of pain relief is speculated: after a local anesthetic is injected in the narrow cavity covered with dense ligaments, the volume of fluid slightly spreads the joint space and improves the joint dysfunction to normal, as well as reduces sensitivity of the nociceptors in the ligaments.

5.2.1.3 Which Is More Effective, Injection into the Posterior Ligamentous Region or the Posterior Nerve Branch?

There are some people who assume that the effect of an SIJ injection originates from injecting local anesthetic into the lateral branch of the sacral nerve [5]. However, Honda et al. [6] showed that for patients with SIJ disorder, radio frequency thermocoagulation into the posterior sacroiliac ligament was more effective than into the posterior lateral branch of the sacral nerves, both immediately after the treatment and 1 month later (Fig. 5.4a–c). This result indicates that pain origin in most patients with SIJ disorder should be into the posterior sacroiliac ligament.

5.2.1.4 Pre-injection Test

MRI

In order to detect the presence or absence of a tumor, abscess, fresh compression fracture, disc herniation, or lumbar spinal stenosis before an injection, an MRI of the lumbar or pelvic region is useful.

Blood Test

For excluding severe diseases, a check for blood sedimentation, CRP, calcium (Ca), phosphorus (P), and alkaline phosphatase (ALP) is necessary.

5.2.1.5 Complications Resulting from Injections

When using the injection technique described previously, there is little possibility that the injection needle will be inserted into the pelvic cavity and the peri-articular injection will cause severe injuries to blood vessels and nerves because essential vessels and nerves are not situated in the posterior ligamentous region.

If a patient complains of (1) numbness of the mouth or tongue, (2) dizziness, (3) ringing in the ears, etc. after injection, there is a possibility of local anesthetic

Fig. 5.4 Thermocoagulation method. (**a**) Device and thermocoagulation conditions. Device: thermocoagulation of a 22 G needle coagulator (produced by Radionics). Stimulation: 50 Hz, less than1.0 V. Formation of thermocoagulation points. (**b**) Diagram of thermocoagulation points: *b-1*: the posterior sacroiliac ligament, *b2*: the posterior lateral branch of the sacral nerves. X: thermocoagulation points. (**c**) Comparison of the efficacy of thermocoagulation in the ligament and at the posterior lateral branch of the sacral nerves. This figure shows that in the early period, thermocoagulation in the ligament should be more effective than that at the posterior lateral nerve branches. The data indicates a higher possibility that the pain origin is in the ligamentous area, rather than the posterior lateral nerve branches. (Provided by Dr. Junya Hanakita, Spinal Disorders Center of Fujieda Heisei Memorial Hospital)

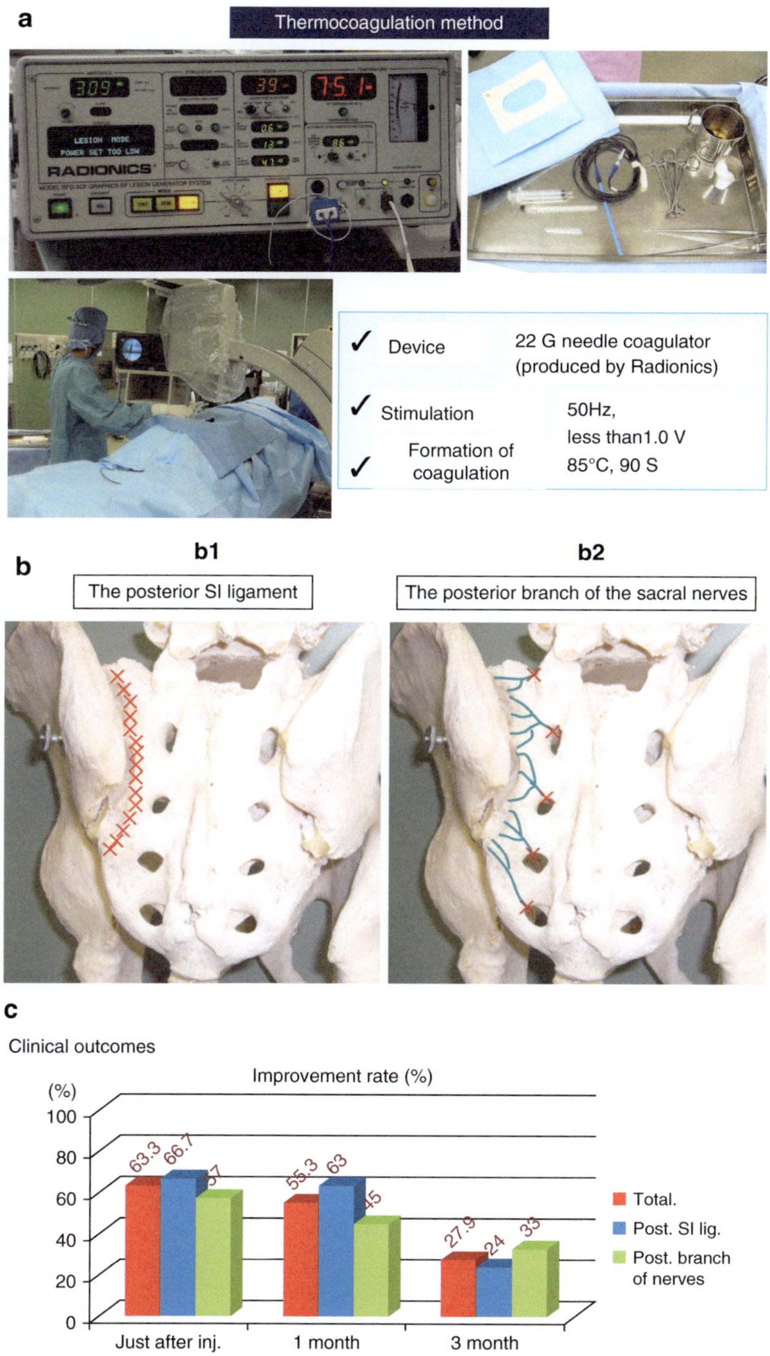
a
Thermocoagulation method
RADIONICS
LESION MODE
POWER SET TOO LOW
Device
22 G needle coagulator (produced by Radionics)
Stimulation
50Hz,
less than1.0 V
Formation of coagulation
85°C, 90 S
b
b1
The posterior SI ligament
b2
The posterior branch of the sacral nerves
c
Clinical outcomes
Improvement rate (%)
(%)
100
80
60
40
20
0
63.3
66.7
57
55.3
63
45
27.9
24
33
Just after inj.
1 month
3 month
Total.
Post. SI lig.
Post. branch of nerves

poisoning. In the event of local anesthetic poisoning, give the patient an intravenous drip with oxygen inhalation, in order to promptly expel the local anesthetic outside the body. We have had some patients who complain of dizziness after an injection. However, in our cases, it was shown to be a reflex induced by pain, and we have not had any patients in a state of shock.

When the insertion site of the needle is suddenly painful and is hot to the touch, an infection should be suspected and a blood test should be performed (the blood should be checked).

For details on the SIJ injection procedure, see Chap. 6 "Manual of Sacroiliac Joint Injection."

5.2.2 **Medications** (Fig. 5.5)

If pain cannot be sufficiently controlled with only an injection, drugs should be used. First, we use nonsteroidal anti-inflammatory drugs (NSAIDs) (including a poultice). As the incidence rate of side effects of NSAIDs, such as gastrointestinal disorder, is between 5 and 15%, we try to use a weak opioid, such as a tramadol combination (Tramset®) or buprenorphine (Norspan Tape®) if sufficient effectiveness is not seen in spite of using two types of NSAIDs (including a suppository). For uncontrollable severe pain, we sometimes use a strong opioid such as morphine hydrochloride. Though morphine hydrochloride has side effects including nausea and constipation, it does not have similar side effects to NSAIDs. Using antiemetic drugs and constipation drugs in combination can decrease these side effects. Using an amount below that causes drowsiness ensures safety. We have not experienced any cases of respiratory disturbance. When a daily dose of around 30–60 mg is used, serious side effects should not usually occur.

Examples of prescriptions for the opioids used are shown below.

Morphine hydrochloride 10 mg tablet: three tablets/day, prochlorperazine (Novamin®); 5 mg tablet: three tablets/day, sennoside (Plesenide®); and 12 mg tablets: two tablets/day.

When morphine hydrochloride is used, many patients express a change in the nature of their pain. If the pain can be controlled, the amount of morphine can be gradually reduced. The drug can be used safely because it does not cause ulcers or other such side effects.

Fig. 5.5 Algorism of medications

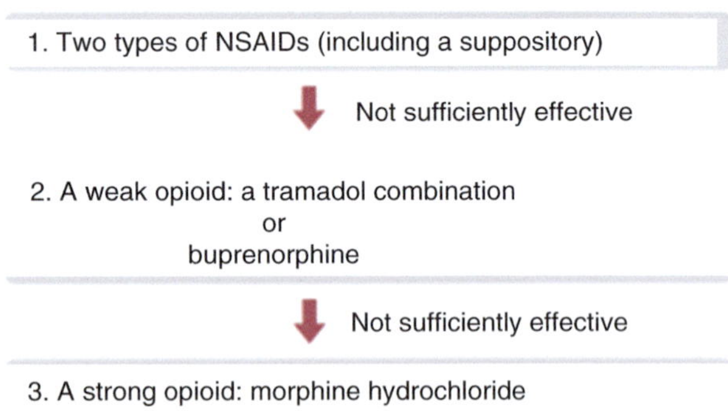

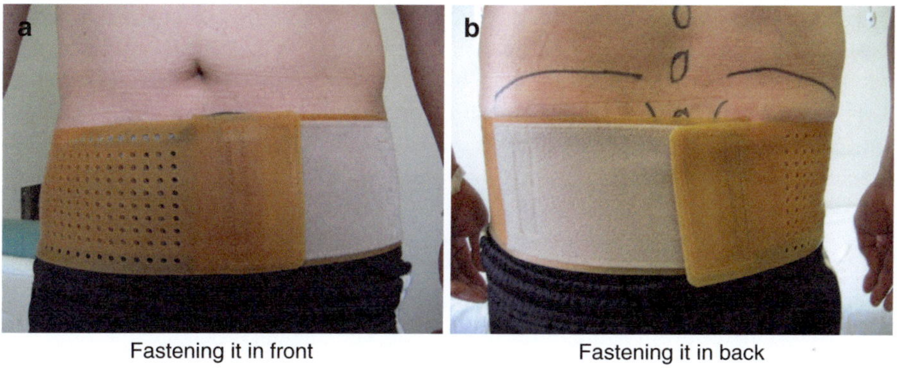

Fig. 5.6 Wearing a rubber pelvic belt. The rubber belt is effective because it does not easily slip. For certain patients, fastening it in the front (**a**) is more effective, or conversely fastening it in the back (**b**) is more effective

5.2.3 Wearing a Rubber Pelvic Belt (Fig. 5.6)

It is unnecessary to fit a patient with a hard brace, like a pelvic brace, when treating SIJ disorder. You can expect sufficient pain relief by having the patient put on a pelvic belt below the iliac crest.

A rubber belt is especially easy to adjust and fasten around the pelvic ring.

As well, you can fasten it in front or in the back. There are some patients with SIJ disorder for whom fastening the rubber belt in front is more effective or conversely fastening it in the back is effective. Thus, patients had better to try it both ways. In addition, the rubber belt has the advantage of not easily slipping.

Key Message: Acute SIJ Disorder Is Effectively Treated by Heating Rather than Cooling

Even for acute SIJ disorder, cooling of the affected area causes pain in many patients. Regardless of the time since onset, pain originating from SIJ disorder is effectively treated by heating rather than cooling. When heating increases pain for certain patients, they may have some form of inflammation in the SIJ.

5.2.4 Arthrokinematic Approach (AKA)-Hakata Method (A Manual Therapy)

A comparative study on the efficacy among physical therapy, chiropractic manipulation, and the provision of educational booklets for treating patients with low back pain concluded that any of these treatments showed only a small effect on low back pain [7].

Even though there is a lack of evidence that manual therapy is superior to other treatments, we would like to introduce an interesting and effective manual therapy which is commonly performed in Japan by many physicians and physical therapists. This therapy is named as arthrokinematic approach (AKA)-Hakata method which was developed in Japan by Setsuo Hakata in1979. This therapy is based on arthrokinematics, articular neurology, and the joint mobilization technique. The manual procedure should improve abnormalities of intra-articular movement of the synovial joint while guiding movement on the joint surface, using four techniques: (1) upward gliding, (2) downward gliding, (3) superior distraction, and (4) inferior distraction (Fig. 5.7). In the manual therapy, the SIJ is gently and slightly moved without developing the arthrostatic reflex in the joint. The manual procedure has obtained good clinical outcomes.

The study by members of the AKA-Hakata method association [8] indicated that the AKA-Hakata method significantly improved pain intensity and the QOL in patients with chronic non-specific low back pain. However, there is a drawback that it takes a long time to master the technique of this method.

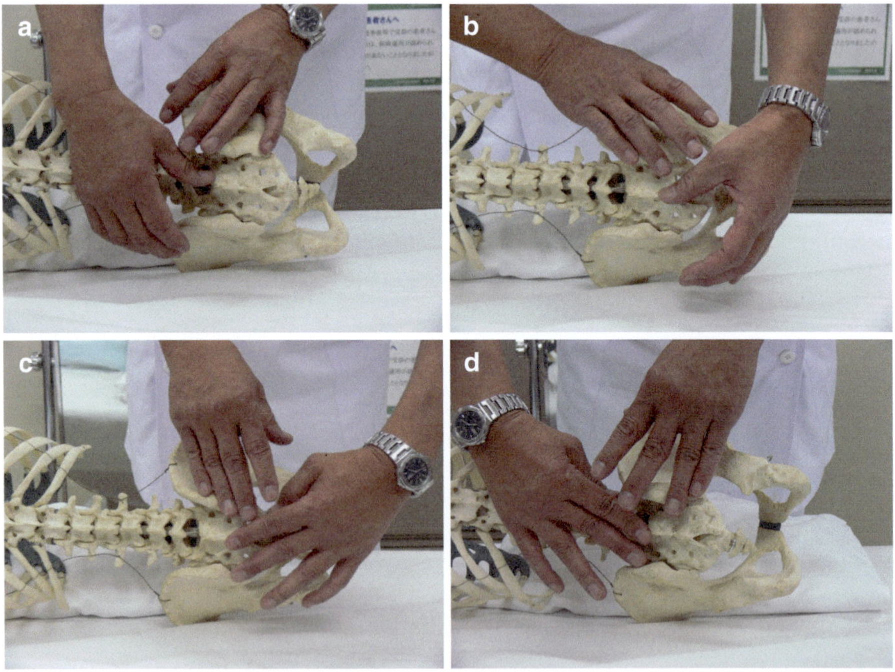

Fig. 5.7 AKA-Hakata method. This manual procedure consists of four techniques. With permission from [23]. (**a**) Upward gliding: while the PSIS and the S1 spinous process are slightly pushed, the cephalad part of the SIJ is separated. (**b**) Downward gliding: while pushing both the ASIS and PSIS and fixing the S3 spinous process with the other thumb, the caudal part of the SIJ is separated. (**c**) Superior distraction: pushing the PSIS and the S1 spinous process induces nutation of the sacrum. (**d**) Inferior distraction: pushing the PSIS and the S3 spinous process induces counter-nutation of the sacrum

5.3 Surgical Treatments

For SIJ pain, conservative therapies such as rest, taking oral analgesics, fixation with a belt, physical therapy, or SIJ injection should mainly be utilized. However, if the pain does not improve using these conservative treatments, SIJ fusion may be the treatment of choice. To date, a number of posterior [9–11], lateral [12, 13], or anterior approaches [14–16] have been attempted; however, sufficient results have not been obtained.

However, in recent years, minimally invasive surgery (MIS) procedures for SIJ fusion, such as the triangular implant system (*iFuse Implant System*) through the lateral approach [17] and the Distraction Interference Arthrodesis with Neurovascular Anticipation (*DIANA*) method through the posterior approach [18], have been developed and become the dominant technique for SIJ arthrodesis used on many patients throughout Europe and the USA with good results.

I would like to briefly describe the recent representative methods for the lateral, posterior, and anterior approaches.

5.3.1 The Lateral Approach: iFuse Implant System (Fig. 5.8)

This system uses a minimally invasive lateral approach with triangular titanium implants and was developed by the SI-Bone, Inc., in the USA. The system is currently the most used approach for fusing and stabilizing the SIJ. The number of patients to have received this approach has already reached more than 25,000 around

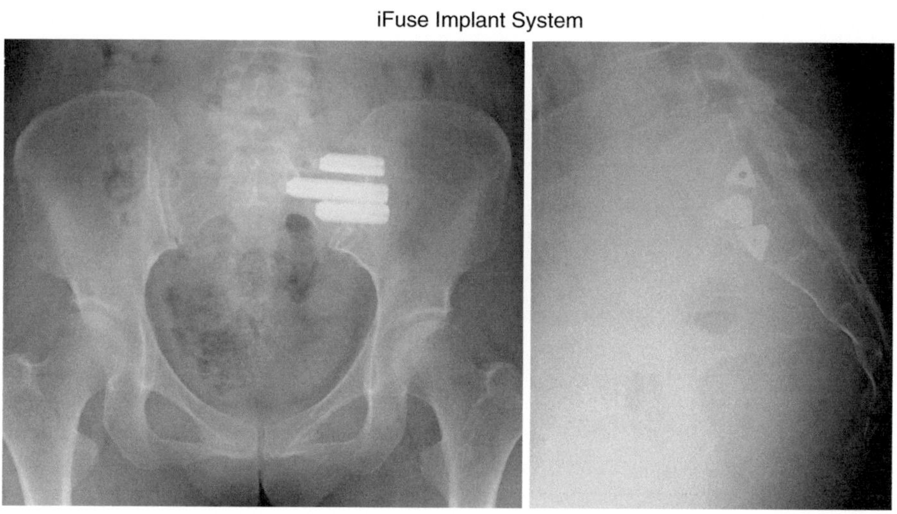

Fig. 5.8 iFuse Implant System. In the majority of patients, three triangular titanium implants are placed into the gluteal region over the S1 using a lateral approach through a short, lateral incision. The most cephalad implant should be seated within the sacral ala above the first neural foramen, the second implant above or adjacent to the S1 foramen, and the third between the S1and S2 foramen

the world and is increasing at a rapid rate. NASS recommends the system as one of the several surgical procedures.

5.3.1.1 Surgical Technique

Under general anesthesia with the patient in the prone position, a lateral short incision (about 3 ~ 4 cm) was made into the gluteal region, positioned over the S1 by lateral fluoroscope imaging. The gluteal fascia and muscle are bluntly dissected to reach the outer table of the ilium. A Steinman pin is placed through the ilium across the SIJ to the center of the sacrum (lateral to the neural foramen) under fluoroscopy. After a soft tissue protector is passed over the pin, the bone is prepared for a triangular channel to receive the implant, using a drill and a triangular broach. Using a pin-guidance system, a total of three implants are placed in the majority of patients.

The most cephalad implant should be seated within the sacral ala above the first neural foramen, as well as the second implant above or adjacent to the S1 foramen and the third between the S1and S2 foramen.

5.3.1.2 Clinical Outcomes

Rudolf's reports of the first 50 patients treated with the iFuse Implant System indicate that patients showed a dramatically early and sustained statistically significant improvement in pain function at 3-, 6-, and 12-month follow-ups [17]. The 5-year outcomes of 17 patients were also favorable as follows [19]. Clinical improvements remained unchanged at 5 years. Pain on VAS improved from 8.3 at baseline to 2.4 at 5 years. Mean ODI score at 5 years was 21.5 (SD 22.7). Patient satisfaction achieved at 12 months was maintained for 5 years (82%). Intra-articular osseous bridging was confirmed in 87% of patients.

Vanaclocha et al. [20] noted the items below in their report of 24 patients treated with the iFuse system.

- Blood loss: mean 58 ml (range, 70–404).
- Time of surgery: mean 48 min (range, 40–65).
- Hospital stay: 1 day in all cases. The average time until returning to work was 47.4 days (range, 30–67).
- Postoperative weight bearing: Neither cane nor crutches are recommended. On the other hand, Rudolf [17] recommended using crutches for a period of time before resuming full activity.

5.3.1.3 Complications

Rudolf L et al. reported ten perioperative complications and a late complication after surgery in 50 patients. The ten perioperative complications included superficial cellulitis in three patients, a deep-soft tissue wound infection in one patient, a large buttock hematoma in two patients, implant penetration into the sacral neural foramen in two patients, compressing the L5 nerve with the first implant due to an unrecognized hemi-sacralized L5 transitional vertebrae in one patient, a non-displaced fracture occurring at the inferior edge of the ilium in one patient, and a late complication of loosened implants in one patient, which occurred 3 years after surgery. On the other hand, the revision rate was reported as 3.5% in a 4-year revision rate (Cher D. Med Device Evid Res 2015.)

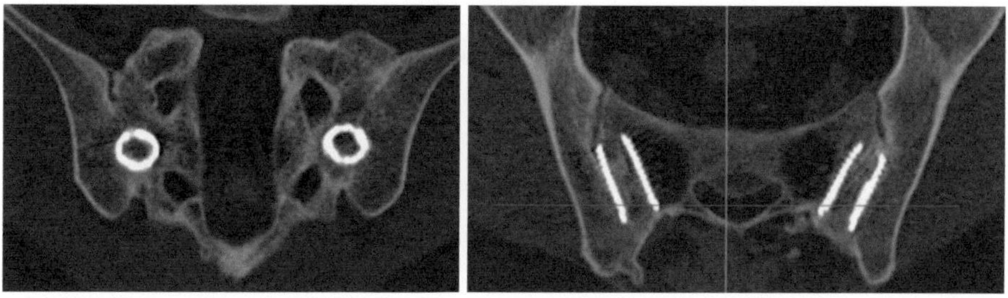

Fig. 5.9 DIANA method. Through a short, posterior, midline incision, the extra-articular recess is identified. The joint is distracted using a herical distraction instrument along the recess after the bone substitute has been packed into the extra-articular recess and joint space. Then, a herical implant is inserted into the hardest part of the iliac bone, following the weight-bearing axis. From Volker Fucks in Germany

This procedure is thought to be immediately beneficial in pain relief and for the functional improvement of SIJ disorder after surgery.

5.3.2 The Posterior Approach: DIANA Method (Fig. 5.9)

This method was introduced by John Stark in 2009 as a revisable surgical method for permanent fusion of the SIJ. The concept of this procedure is the restoring of the joint space by means of controlled distraction followed by expansive bone fusion using the extra-articular recess.

5.3.2.1 Surgical Technique

Through a posterior midline incision (about 4–6 cm), the extra-articular recess is identified, and the bone surfaces are prepared for the bone substitute, using appropriate curettes and a micro burr. The bone substitute, such as beta-tricalcium phosphate, is packed into the recess and space. The joint is distracted using herical distraction instruments which are introduced along within the recess and maintained by a wedge-shaped instrument which is positioned over the guide pin. Then the implant seat is prepared with a reamer, and a herical implant is inserted into the hardest part of the iliac bone, following the weight-bearing axis.

There are not yet reports on the long-term results in patients receiving DIANA.

5.3.2.2 Clinical Outcomes

Endres et al. [21] reported the clinical outcomes of 19 patients receiving DIANA with a mean follow-up of 13.2 months (range, 6–24 months). All patients demonstrated significant improvement in VAS and ODI scores compared to preoperative values. However, the mean VAS score from 8.5 to 6 at the final follow-up demonstrated a 30% improvement in addition to the mean ODI scores showing a 12% improvement from 64.1 to 57. Improvement in pain function would not be so dramatic because all patients had a multilevel lumbar or lumbosacral fusion. The overall fusion rate of SIJ was 78.9% (15/19 joints). They noted the items below in their report:

- Blood loss: <150 ml in all cases.
- Time of surgery: mean 69 min (range, 44–133).
- Hospital stay: mean 7.3 days (range, 3–10).
- Postoperative weight bearing: the partial weight bearing for 6–12 weeks is recommended.

5.3.2.3 Complications

Out of 171 patients, in one case, a sensory L5 radiculitis was caused by too liberally applied bone substitute [18].

5.3.3 The Anterior Approach: Our Anterior SIJ Fusion [22]

5.3.3.1 The Transition of Our Surgical Technique

1999–2000. We performed posterior SIJ fusion using three screws and a bone graft through a hole, which is made for grafting between screws, in three patients. However, considerable pain remained in all three patients and they could not return to their work. We felt that this approach was not enough for treating patients with severe SIJ pain, and we transitioned to the anterior approach.

We felt that the anterior approach had advantages for both sufficient curettage of the joint and performing bone grafting, under direct vision, compared to the lateral or posterior approach. Thus we have mainly performed the SIJ fusion through the anterior approach since 2001.

In the early period, we used an anterior approach to expose the SIJ by separating the iliac muscle from the iliac bone, but later, we changed to a para-rectal approach through the lateral edge of the rectus abdominal muscle.

5.3.3.2 Former Approach (Fig. 5.10)

With the patient in the supine position, while keeping the hip slightly flexed, make an incision along the iliac crest about 10 cm (a). Subperiosteally the iliac muscle is separated from the ilium to reach the anterior surface of the SIJ. Curette the joint space (b), and fix the SIJ with the plate and five screws after grafting with cancellous bone from the ilium (c). At least one of the two screws should be inserted from the sacrum to the ilium to strengthen the fixation of the joint.

5.3.3.3 Current Approach (Fig. 5.11)

The position is the same as that of the former anterior approach. A long longitudinal incision, about 8–10 cm, is made along the lateral border of the rectus abdominal muscle over the line of the SIJ, after identifying the SIJ under fluoroscopy (a). The cavity is deepened in line with the skin incision by cutting the external oblique muscle, internal oblique muscle, and transverse abdominal muscle to reach the peritoneum (b). Extraperitoneally reach the psoas major muscle and the iliac muscle by retracting the peritoneum medially (c). Expose the anterior surface of the SIJ between the two muscles (d). Curette and fix the SIJ in the same manner as the former anterior approach.

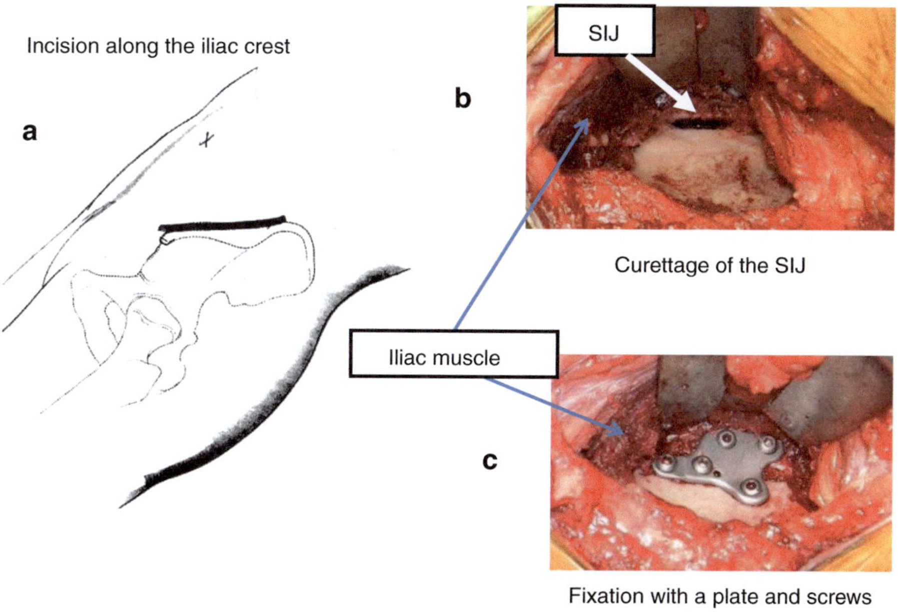

Fig. 5.10 Former anterior approach

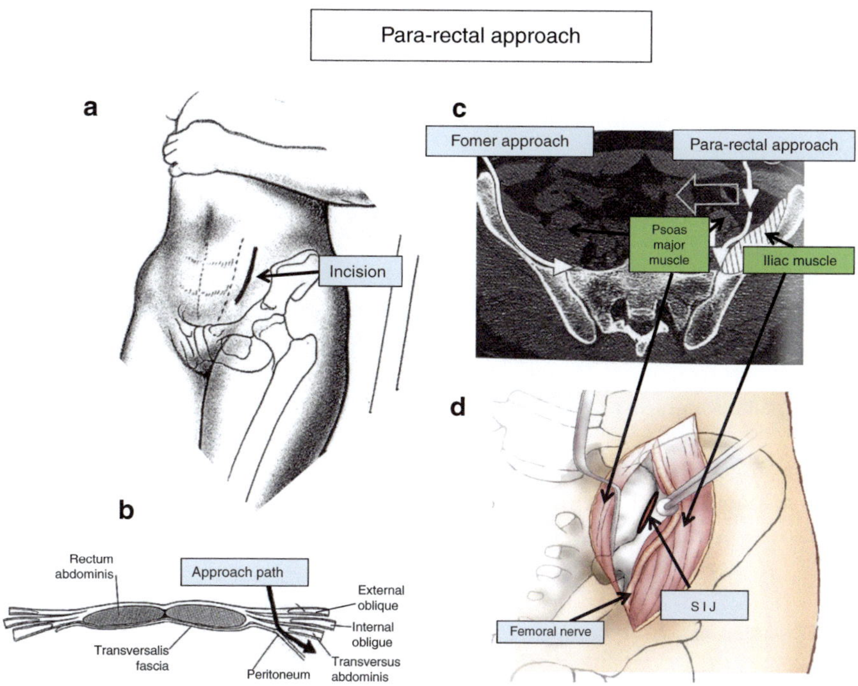

Fig. 5.11 Current anterior approach

5.3.3.4 Clinical Outcomes

We investigated 27 patients who received follow-up for more than 5 years; mean follow-up was 113 months (range, 61–157 months). The group consisted of 21 patients who received a single anterior arthrodesis, 4 patients who required additional posterior fusion, and 2 patients who required pelvic ring arthrodesis due to pain later on the opposite side.

According to the modified MacNab criteria, excellent or good was 21 out of 27 (78%). All 27 patients had bone union of the SIJ on CT. The pain relief scale, VAS for pain, and RDQ also showed significant improvement. VAS: from mean 84.4 (range, 65–95) to mean 26.6 (range, 5–76). RDQ: from mean 21.2 (range, 18–23) to mean 7.2 (range, 0–15). Compared with their preoperative condition, for all patients, sitting time on a chair and walking time improved significantly after the operation with an average of 6.7 min (range, 0–20) to 111.4 min (range, 30–180) and from 10.3 min (range, 0–30) to 81.7 min (range, 1–240), respectively (Fig. 5.12).

- Restricted motion: Most of the 21 patients with a single anterior fusion showed reduction of the flexion-abduction angle of the hip and loss of walking stride, compared to the unaffected side (Fig. 5.13).
- This data indicates that the ROM of the hip may be a combination of the hip joint itself and the SIJ.
- Blood loss: the amount of blood loss was on average 130 (44–271) ml.
- Time of surgery: the length of surgery was on average 190 (150–310) min.
- Hospital stay: the length of hospital stay was 2–3 months among patients with a single anterior SIJ fusion.
- Postoperative weight bearing: partial weight bearing for up to 10–12 weeks should be needed.

5.3.3.5 Complications

- Dislocation of a screw: Dislocation of a screw occurred in three patients.
- Thigh lateral cutaneous neuralgia: Thigh lateral cutaneous neuralgia developed in seven out of a total of 27 patients; among them, six patients underwent the initial anterior method and the other underwent the current method.
- Hematoma formation: Hematoma formation was observed in one patient but it disappeared naturally.

After surgery, pain in the SIJ on the unaffected side appeared in 14 patients, which was able to be controlled in most patients by SIJ injection except for two patients in whom pelvic ring fusion was performed.

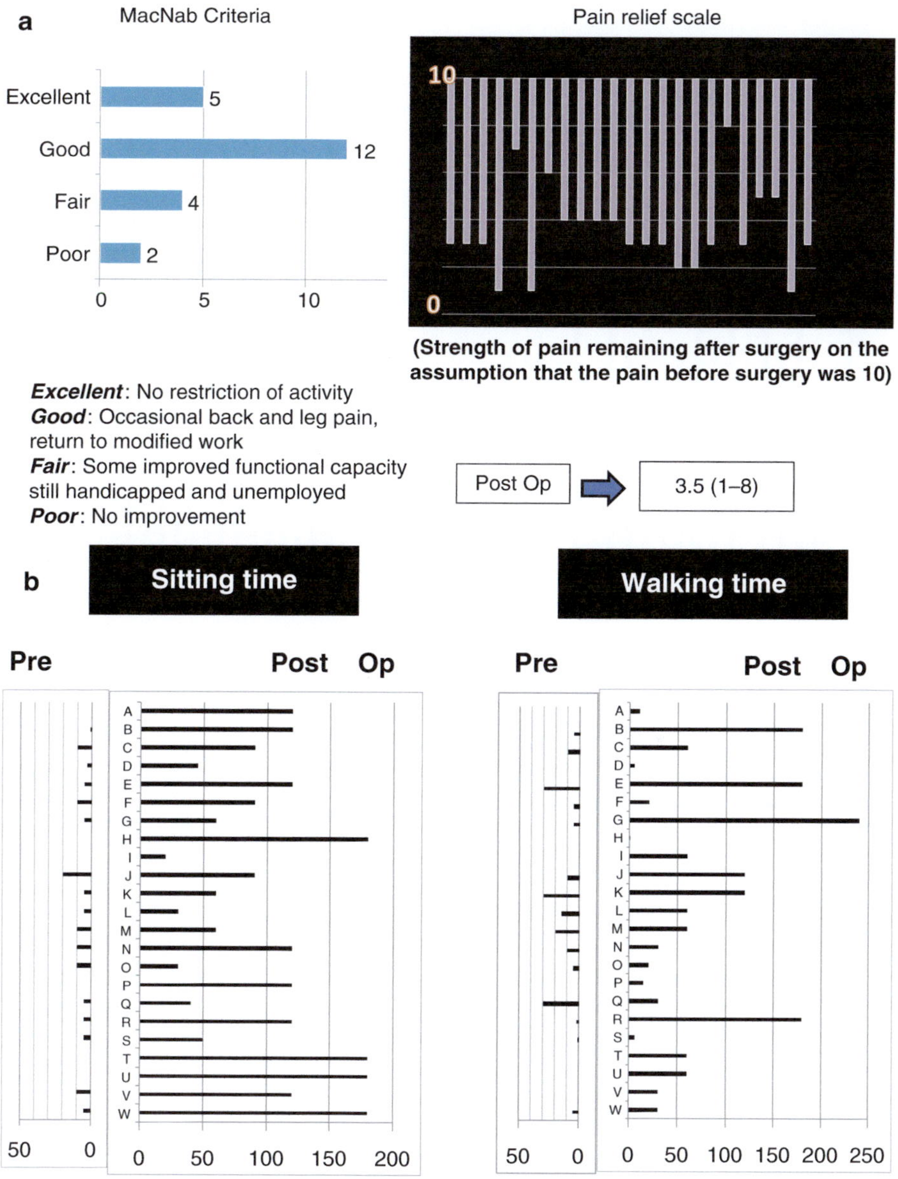

Fig. 5.12 (**a**) Change of MacNab criteria and pain relief scale. (**b**) Change of sitting time and walking time. Time sitting on a chair and time walking improved significantly post-operation

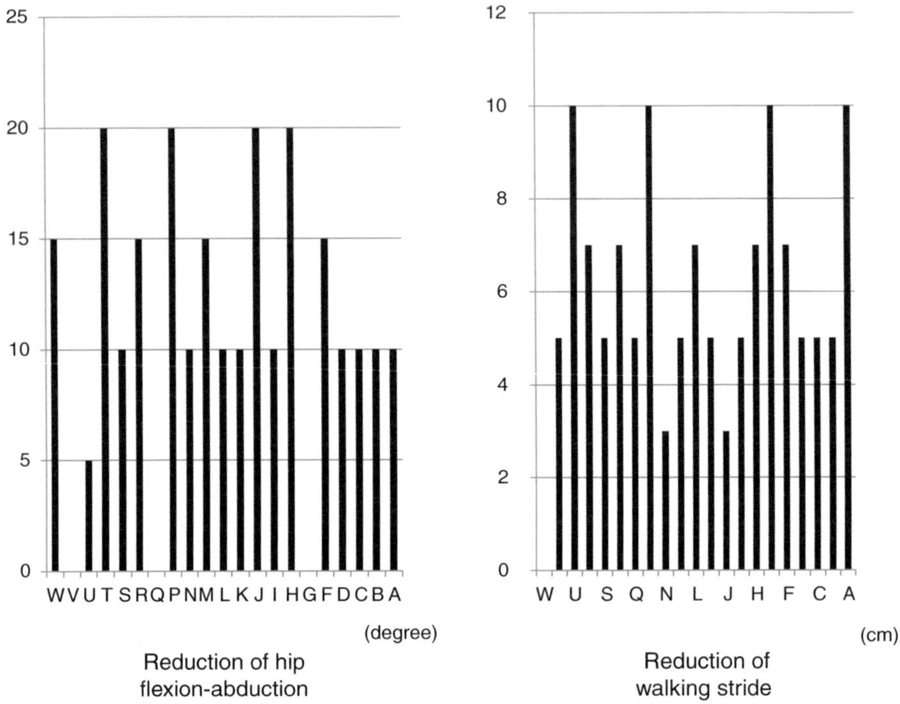

Fig. 5.13 Reduction in hip flexion-abduction and walking stride on the affected side after SIJ fusion. In 21 patients with unilateral SIJ fusion, when compared with the unaffected side, 19 showed a reduction in the flexion-abduction angle of the hip with an average of 11.8° (range, 5–20), and all patients indicated an average of 6.1 cm (range, 3–10) loss in their walking stride

5.3.3.6 The Advantage of Our Anterior Approach

It is undeniable that our anterior arthrodesis is a more morbid procedure than the novel minimally invasive methods. Despite this fact, this arthrodesis has the advantage of curetting and fixing the main load-bearing area of the SIJ under direct vision, which results in definite bony union and stability. Furthermore, we believe that our present anterior approach is an interesting procedure which reaches the SIJ while not separating the iliac muscle from the iliac bone. This approach is essential for managing infections in the SIJ and pseudo-arthrodesis after an MIS or a percutaneous SIJ fusion via the posterior or lateral side; thus surgeons should learn it.

References

1. Murakami E, Tanaka Y, Aizawa T, et al. Effect of peri-articular and intra-articular injections for sacroiliac joint pain: a prospective comparative study. J Orthop Sci. 2007;12:274–80.
2. Lee JH, Lee SH, Song S. Clinical effectiveness of botulinum toxin a compared to a mixture of steroid and local anesthetics as a treatment for sacroiliac joint pain. Pain Med. 2010;11:692–700.

3. Fukui M, Nitta K, Iwashita S, et al. Pulsed radiofrequency applied to sacroiliac ligament for SIJ pain. Pain Clin. 2011;32:1877–80. (in Japanese).
4. Murakami E, Kurosawa D, Aizawa T. Treatment strategy for sacroiliac joint-related pain at or around the posterior superior iliac spine. Clin Neurol Neurosurg. 2018;165:43–6.
5. Bernard TN Jr, Cassidy JD. The sacroiliac joint- pathophysiology, diagnosis, and management. In: Frymoyer JW, editor. The adult spine: principle and practice. New York: Raven Press; 1991. p. 2126–7.
6. Honda F, Hanakita J, Takahasi T, et al. Radiofrequency sacroiliac joint thermocoagulation for sacroiliac syndrome. J Spine Res. 2010;1:445. (in Japanese).
7. Cherkin DC, Deyo RA, Battie M, et al. A comparison of physical therapy, chiropractic manipulation and the provision of educational booklets for treating patients with low back pain. N Engl J Med. 1998;339:1021–9.
8. Kogure A, Kotani K, Katada S, et al. A randomized, single-blind, placebo-controlled study on the efficacy of the arthrokinematic approach-hakata method in patients with chronic nonspecific low back pain. PLoS One. 2015;10(12):e0144325. https://doi.org/10.1371/journal.pone.0144325.
9. Belanger TA, Dall BE. Sacroiliac arthrodesis using a posterior midline fascial splitting approach and pedicle screw instrumentation: a new technique. J Spinal Disord. 2001;14:118–24.
10. Mitchell JI. Surgical treatment of affections of the lumbo-sacral and sacroiliac joints. Surgery. 1938;4:33–43.
11. Waisbrod H, Krainick JU, Gerbershagen HU. Sacroiliac joint arthrodesis for chronic lower back pain. Arch Orthop Trauma Surg. 1987;106:238–40.
12. Giannikas KA, Khan AM, Karski MT, et al. Sacroiliac joint fusion for chronic pain: a simple technique avoiding the use of metal work. Eur Spine J. 2004;13:253–6.
13. Smith-Petersen MN, Rogers WA. End-result study of arthrodesis of the sacro-iliac joint for arthritis-traumatic and non-traumatic. J Bone Joint Surg Am. 1926;8-A:118–36.
14. Avila L Jr. Primary pyogenic infection of the sacro-iliac articulation. A new approach to the joint. Report of seven cases. J Bone Joint Surg Am. 1941;23-A:922–8.
15. Pennal GF, Massiah KA. Nonunion and delayed union of fractures of the Pelvis. Clin Orthop Relat Res. 1980;151:124–9.
16. Rand JA. Anterior sacro-iliac arthrodesis for post-traumatic sacro-iliac arthritis. J Bone Joint Surg Am. 1985;67-A:157–9.
17. Rudolf L. Sacroiliac joint arthrodesis-MIS technique with Titanium implants: repot of the first 50 patients and outcomes. Open Orthop J. 2012;6:495–502.
18. Fucks V, Ruhl B. Distraction arthrodesis of the sacroiliac joint: 2-year results of a descriptive prospective multi-center cohort study in 171 patients. Eur Spine J. 2017;27:194–204. https://doi.org/10.1007/s00586-017-5313-2.
19. Rudolf L, Capobianco R. Five year clinical and radiographic outcomes after minimally invasive sacroiliac joint fusion using triangular implants. Open Orthop J. 2014;8:375–83.
20. Vanaclocha VV, Lópes FV, Pardo MS, et al. Minimally invasive sacroiliac joint arthrodesis: experience in a prospective series with 24 patients. J Spine. 2014;3(5). https://doi.org/10.1155/2013/536128.
21. Endres S, Ludwig E. Outcome of distraction interference arthrodesis of the sacroiliac joint for sacroiliac arthritis. Indian J Orthop. 2013;47:437–42.
22. Murakami E, Kurosawa D, Aizawa T. Sacroiliac joint arthrodesis for chronic sacroiliac joint pain—a technique of anterior approach and clinical outcomes with minimum 5-year follow up. Neurosurg Spine. https://doi.org/10.3171/2018.1.SPINE17115.
23. Murakami E. Sacroiliac joint pain: undiagnosed low back pain. Tokyo: Nankodo; 2012. (in Japanese).

Manual for Sacroiliac Joint Injections

6

Abstract

- First, a peri-articular injection should be performed.
- The peri-articular injection under fluoroscopic guidance is necessary in order to be precisely performed and confirm pain relief.
- The bedside peri-articular injection without fluoroscopy is a simple and useful method.
- A needle insertion into the posterior ligamentous areas of the SIJ from the cranial side of the PSIS toward the caudal side is the safest procedure.
- Do not be nervous about the depth of the needle for insertion. It is very important to hunt for the area where the familiar pain is induced by needle insertion.
- An injection only into the sections where the patient says "right there" or "this is my pain" by needle insertion should be performed and should be effective.
- As for intra-articular SIJ injections, Kurosawa's technique via the middle portion of the joint can be recommended owing to its high success rate.

6.1 The Peri-Articular Injection Under Fluoroscopic Guidance [1]

For peri-articular injections, an injection needle is aimed at the posterior ligamentous areas of the SIJ (Fig. 6.1a, b).

The injection into the posterior ligamentous region is not dangerous!

In the posterior ligamentous region of the SIJ, no important blood vessels or nerves are found, so there is no worry of severe nerve or blood vessel damage from an injection needle.

E. Murakami, *Sacroiliac Joint Disorder*,
https://doi.org/10.1007/978-981-13-1807-8_6

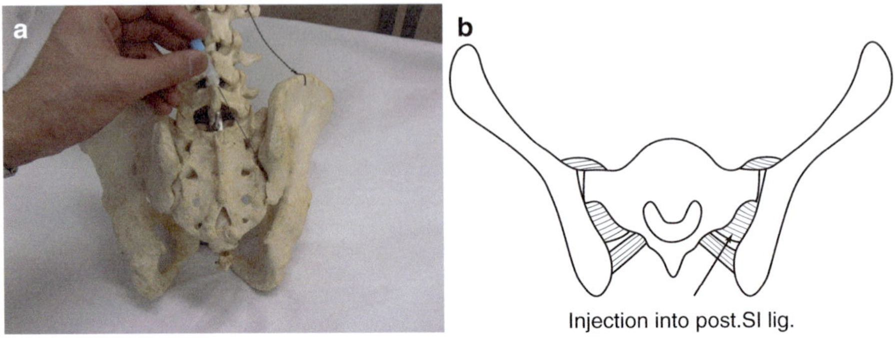

Fig. 6.1 Injection procedure. With permission from [7]. (**a**) A needle insertion on a pelvic specimen: insert the needle into the cleft between the sacrum and the iliac bone. (**b**) Injection into the ligaments behind the joint: for the sacroiliac joint injection, local anesthetic is injected not into the joint cavity but into the posterior ligaments which are considered to be a source of pain in many cases

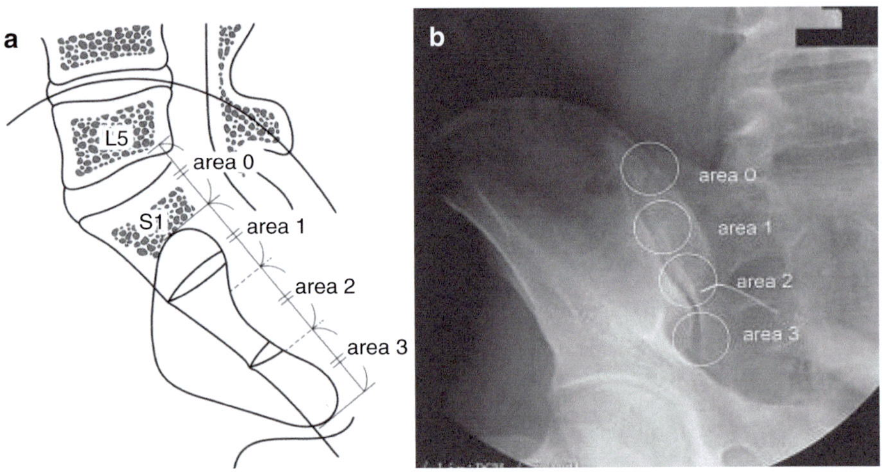

Fig. 6.2 We divide the posterior of the sacroiliac joint into four sections which include three sections in the compartment of ligaments behind the joint cavity (Area 1–3) and one section on the cranial side (Area 0). With permission from [7] ((**a**) Lateral view (**b**) AP view)

6.1.1 Sections Designated for an Injection

The extra-posterior area of the SIJ is divided into four equal sections, which are designated as Areas 0–3. Although Area 0 comprises the cranial portion of the joint, this area is included as an injection target because it contains the posterior ligaments of the SIJ. Areas 1 and 2 contain the interosseous ligaments and the posterior sacroiliac ligament, and Area 3 contains the posterior ligament, a part of the long posterior sacroiliac ligament and the sacrotuberous ligament (Fig. 6.2).

A peri-articular injection is much easier to administer than an intra-articular injection, and you should be able to successfully perform it under fluoroscopy [1].

A 23-gauge needle is inserted into the four sections to confirm the origin of pain.

The region where the needle should be inserted is the ligament region behind the joint cavity as shown in Fig. 6.3. The region is covered by the posterior sacroiliac ligament and the deep interosseous sacroiliac ligament and shows the anatomical features illustrated below [1–4] (Fig. 6.4).

1. Area 0: Chiefly, the superficial layer is the lumbar fascia, and the deep layer is covered by the ligament connecting the L5, the sacrum, and the iliac bone.
2. Area 1: The sacrum and the iliac bone are tightly bound by the interosseous sacroiliac ligament.
3. Area 2: The deep layer is part of the interosseous sacroiliac ligament, and the superficial layer is covered by the posterior sacroiliac ligament. In this section, the area caudal to the lower end of PSIS is the proper site for inserting the needle, due to a lack of bony wall.
4. Area 3: This area contains the posterior sacroiliac and sacroiliac ligament.

The anatomy of the areas where the injection needle penetrates is as follows (Fig. 6.5): The surface layer into which the injection needle is inserted includes the thoracolumbar fascia attaching to the ilium and the erector spinae muscles which are attached to the sacrum (Fig. 6.5a). In the middle layer, there is a part of the multifidus muscles and the posterior sacroiliac ligament (Fig. 6.5b). In the deep layer, the posterior sacroiliac ligament, the interosseous sacroiliac ligament, and the sacrotuberous ligament connect the sacrum and ilium (Fig. 6.5c).

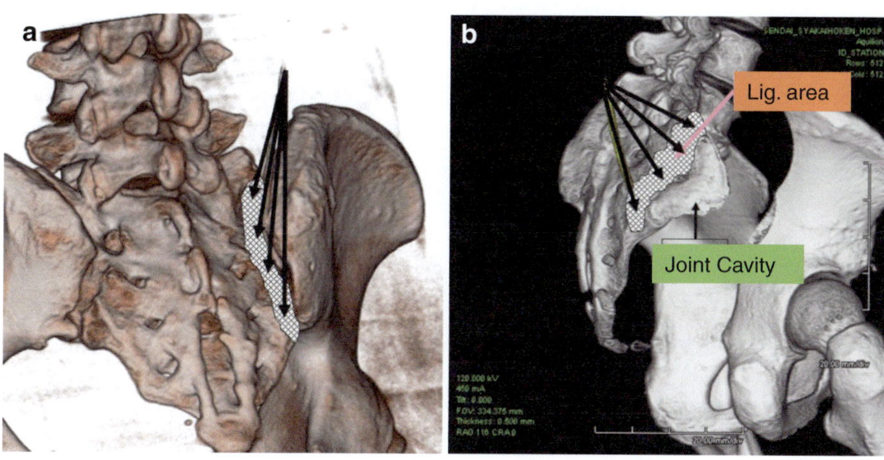

Fig. 6.3 The posterior ligamentous region into which the needle is inserted. With permission from [7]. (**a**) Oblique view. (**b**) Lateral view. Insert an injection needle into the four sections behind the joint cavity

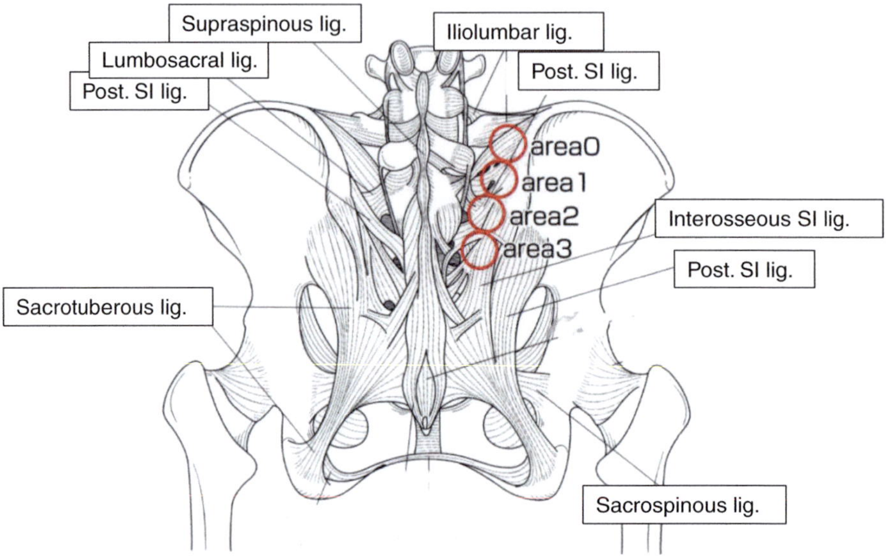

Fig. 6.4 The anatomy of the four sections to be injected. With permission from [7]. Area 0 is mainly comprised of part of the lumbosacral ligament and the upper part of the sacroiliac ligament. Areas 1 and 2 are made up of (=comprised of) the interosseous sacroiliac ligament and the posterior sacroiliac ligament. In Area 3, the posterior sacroiliac ligament and the sacroiliac ligament attach to the iliac and sacrum

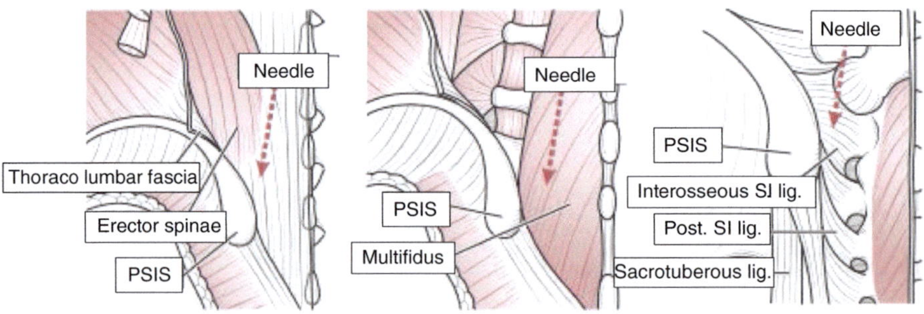

Fig. 6.5 The anatomy of the areas that an injection needle penetrates. With permission from [7]. (**a**) Surface layer: the thoracolumbar fascia in the ilium and the spinal column are attached to the sacrum. (**b**) Intermediate layer: a portion of the multifidus and posterior sacroiliac ligament covers the joint space. (**c**) Deep layer: the posterior sacroiliac ligament, the interosseous sacroiliac ligament, and the sacrotuberous ligament tightly connect the sacrum and the iliac bone

6.1.2 Supplies/Necessary Items for an Injection (Fig. 6.6)

6.1.2.1 Insertion Needle

A 90-mm 23-gauge spinal needle (or a 60-mm 23-gauge needle) is used on occasion.

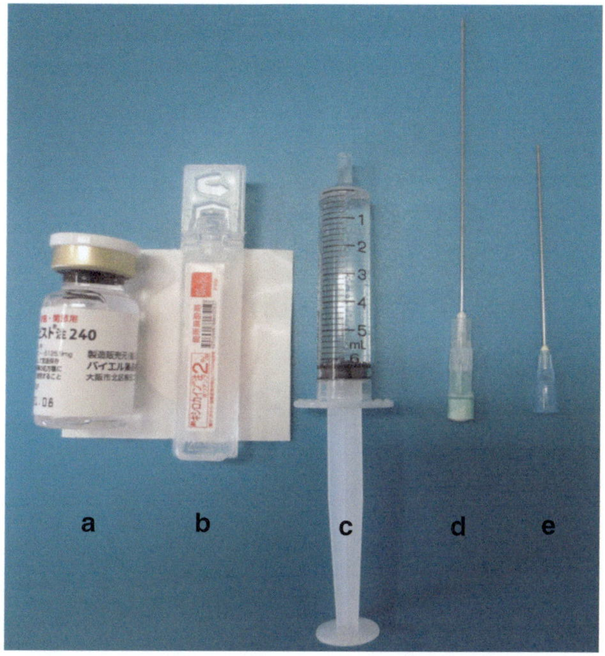

Fig. 6.6 Items to be used in an injection under fluoroscopy. (**a**) Omnipark® 240 (contrast medium), (**b**) 2% lidocaine, (**c**) 5 ml syringe, (**d**) a 90-mm 23-gauge spinal needle, (**e**) a 60-mm 23-gauge needle

6.1.2.2 A Syringe

A 5 ml syringe, because it is better suited to feel resistance than a 10 ml syringe when injecting the local anesthetic.

6.1.2.3 The Local Anesthetic

In order to confirm the extent to which the local anesthetic has spread, a mixture of 2% lidocaine and a contrast medium (mixture ratio 1:1) is used. We do not usually use a steroid such as prednisolone. The reason for this is that most pain from the SIJ is caused by dysfunction, not by inflammation. Hence, a steroid will not be effective in dysfunction of the joint.

6.1.3 Procedure

First, the skin is sterilized, and the patient lies in a prone oblique position with the affected side down on a fluoroscopic table. While the angle of the gantry is parallel to the L5/S1 disc, the patient is rotated so as much of the target section can be clearly detected as possible (Fig. 6.7a).

A 90-mm 23-gauge spinal needle is inserted into each section. At the point where a section is most clearly detected, insert the needle directly aiming for the center of the section. The midway point between the PSIS and the spinous process is often an appropriate insertion point.

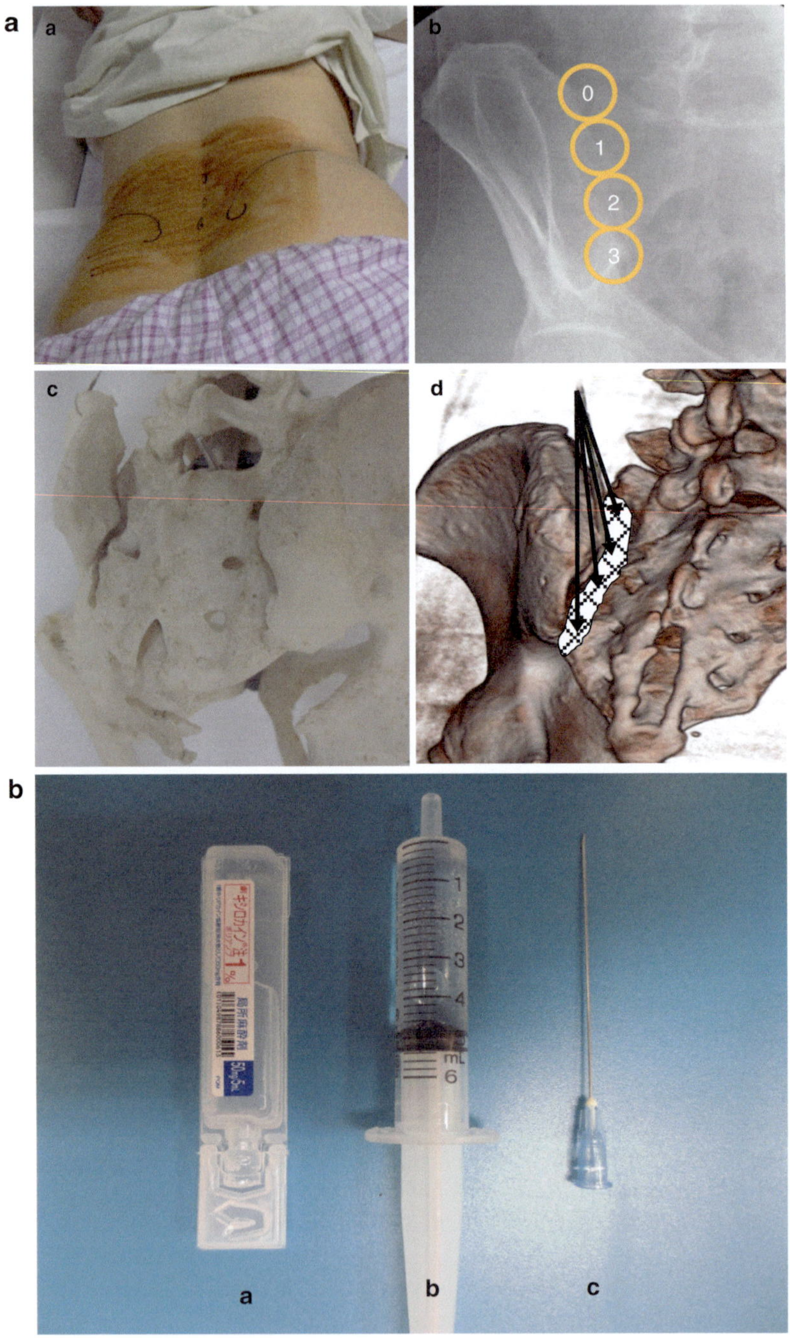

Fig. 6.7 (**a**) The position of the patient on the fluoroscopic table. *a*: The patient lies in a prone oblique position with the affected side down. *b*: The posterior peri-articular area of SIJ is divided into four sections (Areas 0–3). *c*: Bone model in a prone oblique position. *d*: Diagram of needle insertions. (**b**) Items for a simple peri-articular injection under fluoroscopy. *a*: 1% lidocaine, *b*: 5 ml syringe, *c*: a 60-mm 23-gauge needle

Only into sections where familiar pain develops when a needle is inserted, a mixture of 2% lidocaine and a contrast medium (mixture ratio 1:1, total 2 ml) is injected into the posterior ligamentous area while confirming that the solution does not spread to other regions. We can commonly reproduce familiar pain in two or three sections when a needle is inserted.

In order to confirm that the solution anesthetizes only the injected section, it is necessary to use a contrast medium.

However, when administering an injection only for the purpose of obtaining clinical effectiveness, rather than data collection, a solution of 1% lidocaine without a contrast medium is sufficient (Fig. 6.7b).

When the needle is inserted, only normal stinging pain occurs in areas which are not a source of pain. If the area is a source of pain, strong pain occurs when stimulated. It is supposed that in areas where pain originates, there is an increase of chemical mediators such as substance P and CGRP.

6.1.4 Volume of Local Anesthetic to Be Injected

When local anesthetic is injected into a section covered with thick ligaments, it easily leaks out of the compartment (Fig. 6.8). For each section, it is considered that 0.5–1 ml may be the maximum volume that does not cause spreading to the other sections.

6.1.5 Check the Depth of the Injection Needle

The counter-oblique view with the affected side up is useful for detecting the depth of the injection needle.

Ideally, the position of the needle tip is at a depth of 0.5–1.0 cm posteriorly from the joint space.

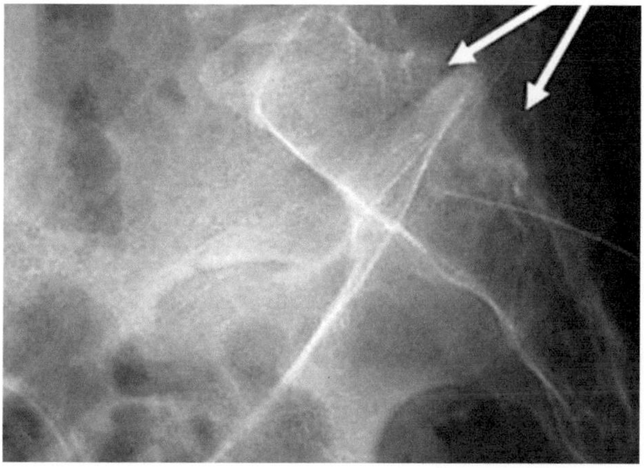

Fig. 6.8 Leakage of local anesthetic. If you inject more than 1 ml of local anesthetic, the liquid can easily leak out of the compartment (arrow). With permission from [7]

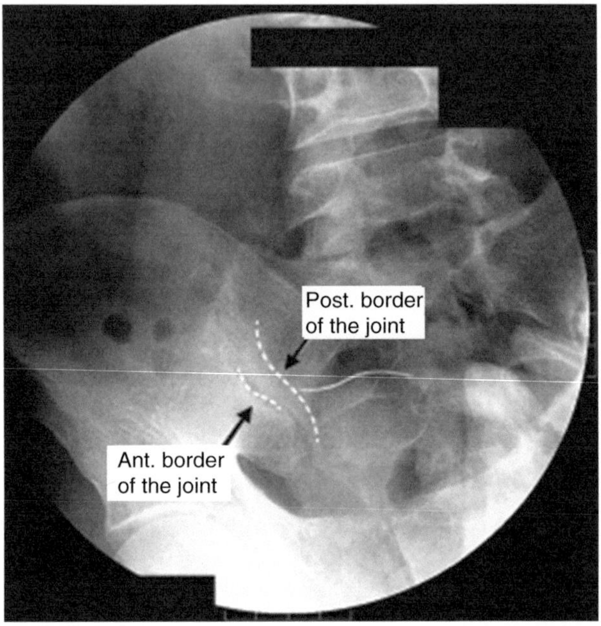

Fig. 6.9 The counter-oblique view is useful for checking the needle tip. The distance between the posterior edge of the joint cavity and the needle tip can be confirmed from the counter-oblique view with the affected side up. With permission from [7]

The counter-oblique view with the affected side up is useful for detecting the distance between the posterior edge of the joint cavity and the tip of the needle. The angle from which the above distance is shown at its longest indicates the actual distance (Fig. 6.9).

In fact, there is no need to be nervous about the depth of the needle, because you can obtain sufficient effect by injecting the local anesthetic at the depth where a patient's familiar pain can be reproduced.

6.1.6 Actual Injection Procedure

For Area 0 and Area 1, the same skin penetration from the cranial side should be performed. Similarly, for Area 2 and Area 3, the skin penetration by 23-G spinal needle is needed (Fig. 6.10).

6.1.6.1 Injection into Area 0

Area 0 is the gap above the upper joint cavity of the sacrum and ilium, which includes a part of the iliolumbar ligament and the area where the ligaments attach to the bones.

If pain is reproduced by needle stimulation, the injection into Area 0 is performed. In Area 0, the familiar pain is often reproduced in the gap between the sacrum and ilium and near the upper outward edges of the sacrum or the ilium (Fig. 6.11). In this section there is a possibility of the needle penetrating the pelvic cavity as there is no osseous wall in Area 0. Care is required for injections into Area 0.

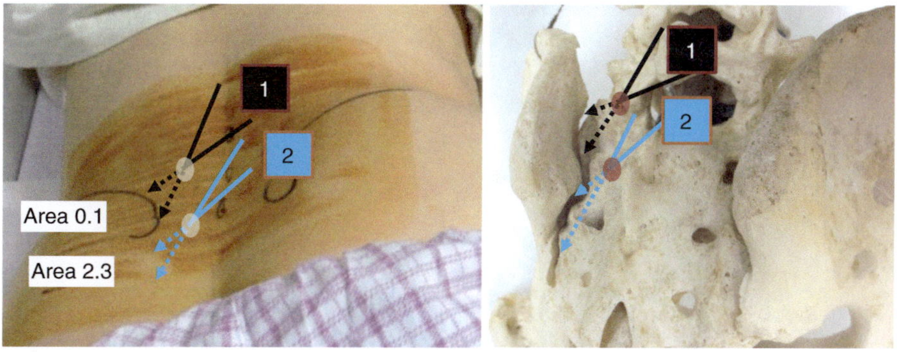

Fig. 6.10 Two skin punctures for needle insertion into four sections are generally necessary

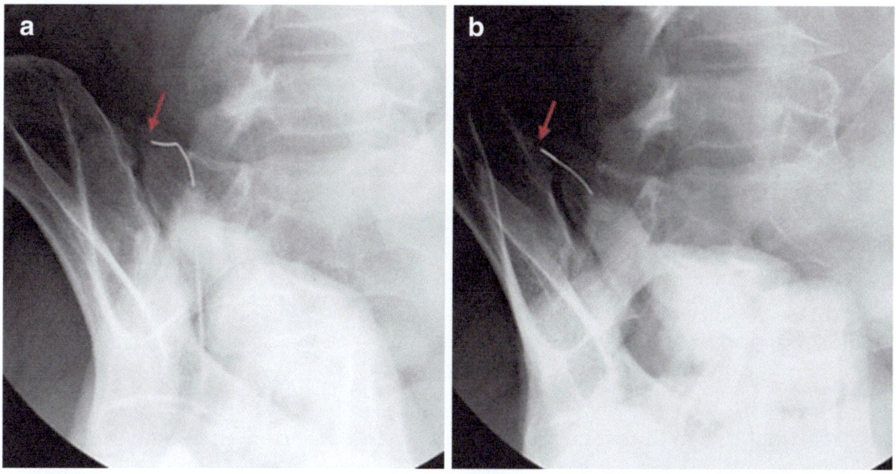

Fig. 6.11 Injection into Area 0. With permission from [7]. (**a**) Injection near the upper outward edge of the sacrum. (**b**) Injection near the upper outward edge of the ilium. The red arrow indicates the tip of the needle. Care is required for injections into Area 0 for a low risk of penetration into the pelvic cavity

6.1.6.2 Injection into Area 1

Area 1 is deep below the skin where the ilium is trapped. It is necessary to insert a needle from the cranial side with the patient in a more oblique position to prevent the ilium from covering Area 1. Directly insert the 90-mm 23-gauge spinal needle, aiming at the center of the compartment (Fig. 6.12a). The distance between the tip of the needle and the posterior border of the SIJ is confirmed by the counter-oblique view (Fig. 6.12b). As it is often difficult to access this area with the tip of the needle, local anesthetic can be injected as long as pain reproduction has been confirmed.

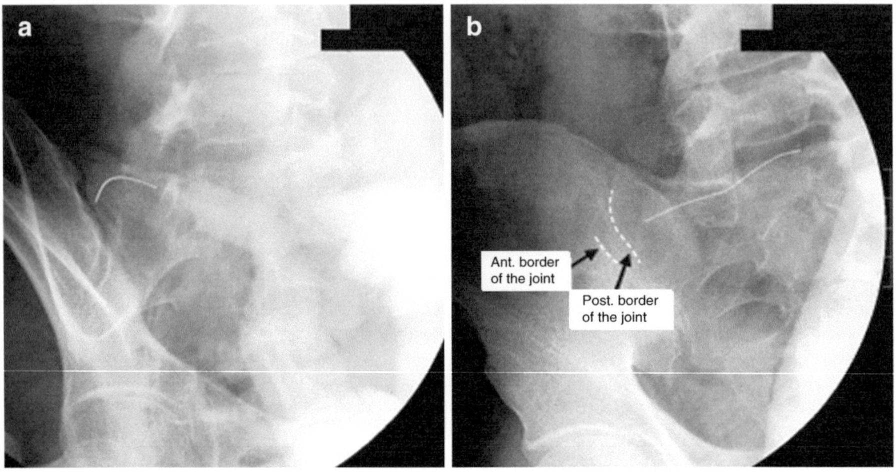

Fig. 6.12 Injection into Area 1. With permission from [7]. (**a**) Oblique view with patient's affected side down. (**b**) Counter-oblique view: the tip of the needle can be confirmed. It is often difficult to access to the posterior border of the SIJ with the tip of the needle

Key Message: Tips for Insertion into Area 1

In some cases, it is necessary to put the patient in a severely oblique position with the painful side down to insert the needle into Area 1 due to the prominence of the ilium. However, as the patient is positioned more obliquely, the insertion point becomes closer to the center of the trunk, making it more difficult to insert the needle. In such cases, the needle must travel a long distance to reach the area.

I would like to introduce some tips for needle insertion in such a case.

First, 1–2 cm inside of the ilium should be determined as the insertion point.

After the needle is inserted roughly 1 cm (Fig. 6.13a), sliding the skin medially toward the sacrum while holding the needle firmly allows the needle to curve (Fig. 6.13b). Then, while adjusting the position, advance the curving needle to the target area, passing through the inner edge of the ilium (Fig. 6.13c).

Using this insertion method, the needle can reach the target region at a relatively short distance from the body surface.

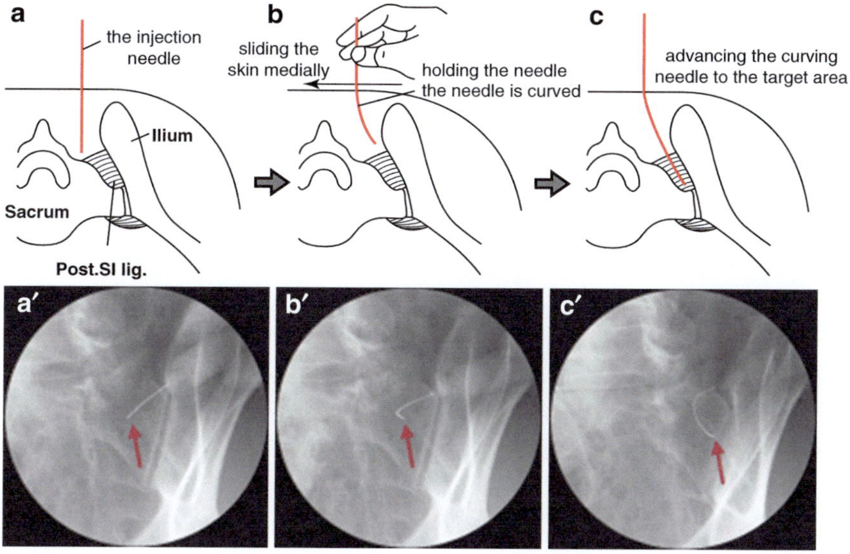

Fig. 6.13 Tips for insertion into Area 1. With permission from [7]. (**a**) A slight insertion of the needle. (**b**) Sliding the skin while holding the needle in order to curve the needle. (**c**) Advancing the curving needle to the target area. With permission from [7]

Table 6.1 Pain reproducibility of each section (out of 25 cases)

Area 0: 1 case
Area 1: 8 cases
Area 2: 19 cases
Area 3: 6 cases

6.1.6.3 Injection into Area 2

As described in Table 6.1, based on data that the central compartment of the joint space (Area 2) had the highest rate of pain reproducibility in four sections, it is likely most efficient to first aim at Area 2.

Fortunately, in many cases, the intersection of the lower end of the PSIS and the joint space is located near the center of Area 2.

As there is no bony wall in many cases, it is easy to first aim at the lower end of the PSIS (Fig. 6.14a) with a needle (90-mm 23-gauge spinal needle). And, after pain is reproduced, having confirmed the distance between the posterior border of the

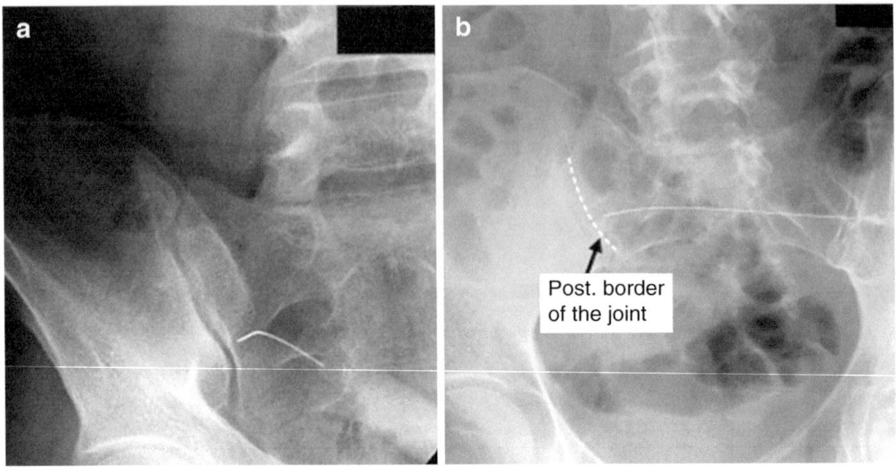

Fig. 6.14 A needle insertion into Area 2. (**a**) Oblique view. (**b**) Counter-oblique view with the affected side down; confirm the depth of the needle tip. With permission from [7]

joint cavity and the needle tip from the counter-oblique view with the patient's affected side up (Fig. 6.14b), inject 0.5–1 ml of 1% lidocaine.

6.1.6.4 Injection into Area 3

Next, inject into Area 3 caudally using the same insertion point as Area 2. This area is the lower part of the SIJ, which includes origin of the posterior sacroiliac ligament and sacrotuberous ligament (Fig. 6.15a). A needle is inserted in the lower part of the joint space as an indicator. Stimulate the lower part of the joint space and the attachment area of the ligament to the sacrum (Fig. 6.15b) and to the ilium (Fig. 6.15c) with the needle tip. If pain is reproduced, inject approximately 1 ml of 1% lidocaine.

6.1.7 Referred Pain Area of Each Section

We examined referred pain for each section; the results indicated that there was a tendency for Areas 0 and 1 to induce referred pain from the upper gluteal to the groin area and for Areas 2 and 3 to develop pain from the lower gluteal to the posterior thigh [2] (Figs. 6.16, 6.17, 6.18, and 6.19).

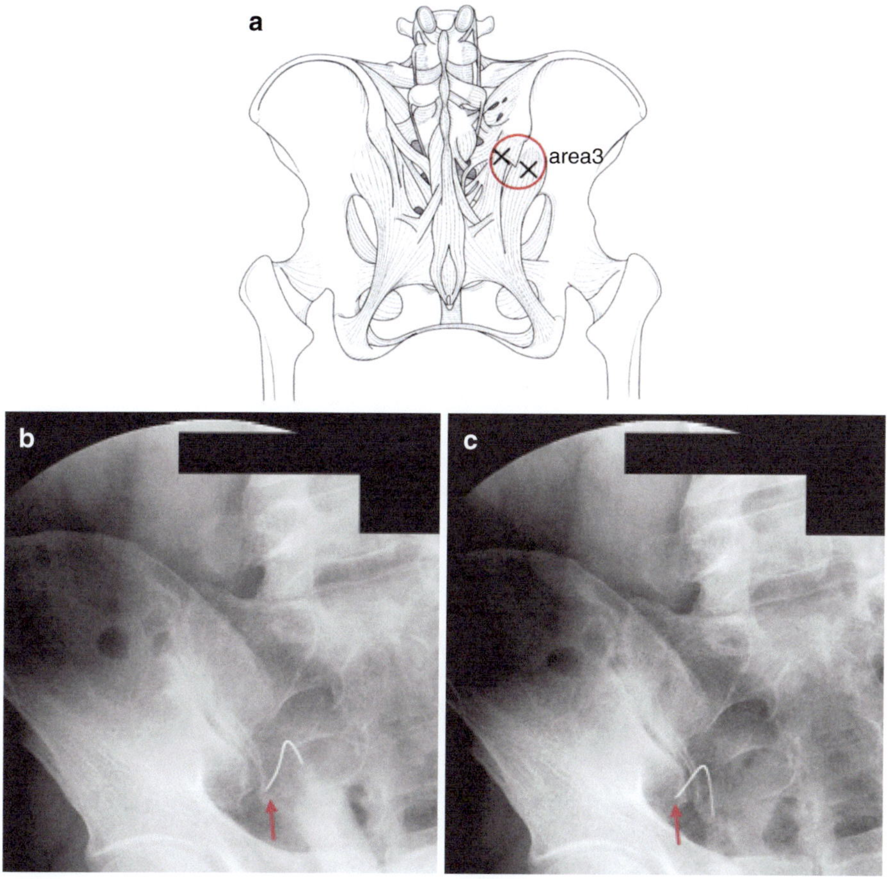

Fig. 6.15 Anatomy of Area 3 and insertion of the needle. (**a**) Posterior sacroiliac ligament and sacrotuberous ligament attached to the sacrum and the ilium. (**b**) Insertion to sacral side. (**c**) Insertion to iliac side. In the figure, × indicates the injection site; the red arrows of (**b**) and (**c**) indicate the tip of the needle. With permission from [7]

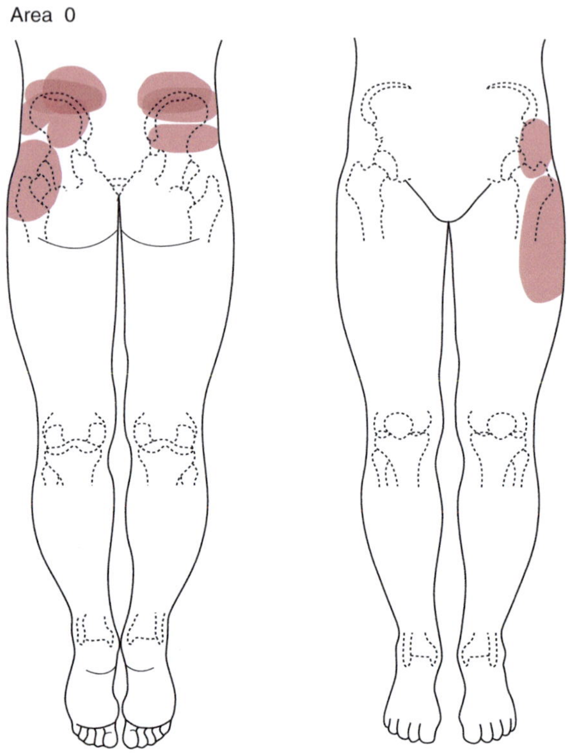

Fig. 6.16 Area 0-related pain. There is related pain from the iliac crest down the side and front of the thigh. With permission from [7]

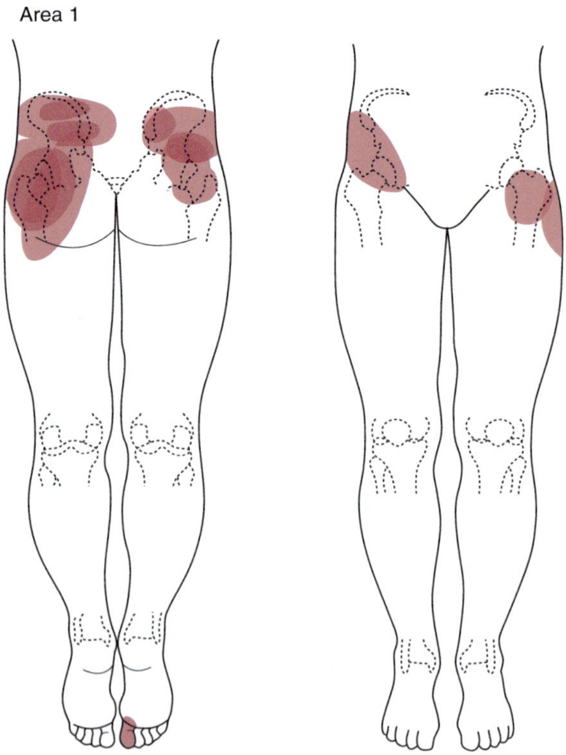

Fig. 6.17 Area 1-related pain. There is related pain from the buttocks to the groin. With permission from [7]

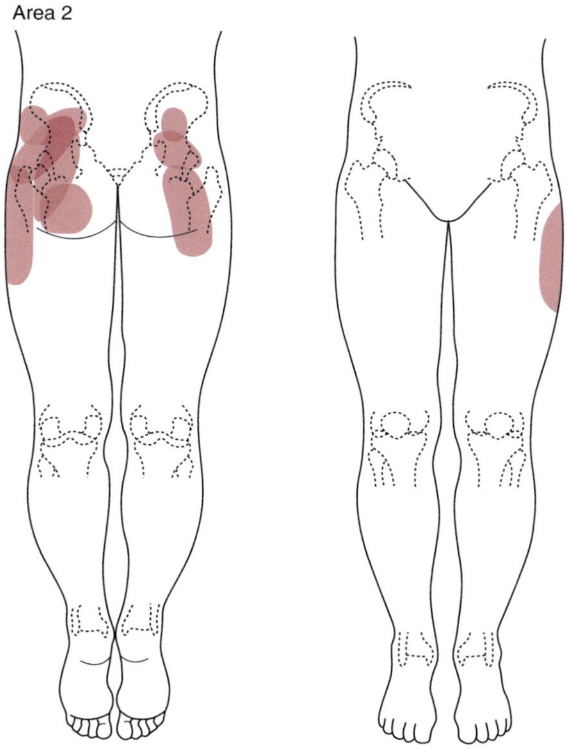

Fig. 6.18 Area 2-related pain. There is related pain from the buttocks to the back of the thigh. With permission from [7]

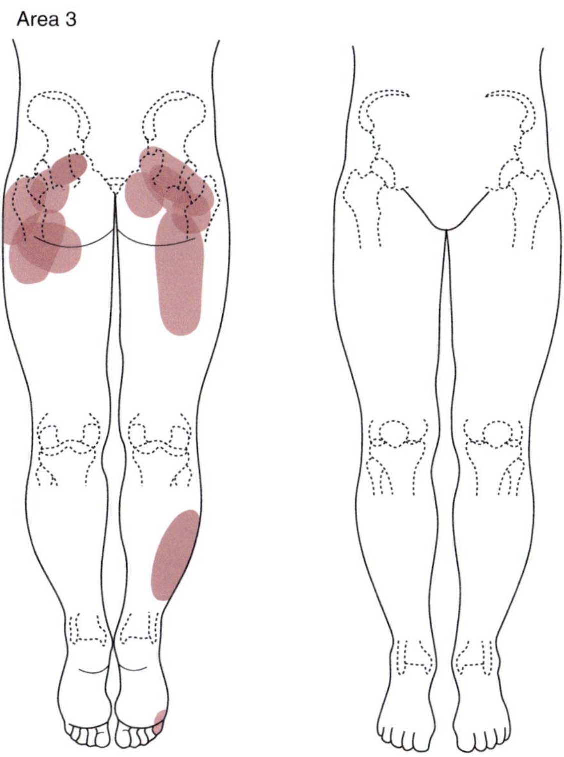

Fig. 6.19 Area 3-related pain. There is related pain from the lower part of the buttock to the back of the thigh. With permission from [7]

Key Message: Summary of Referred Pain Areas from the Four Sections
To summarize the referred pain areas from the four sections, most groin pain is referred from Areas 0 and 1, whereas most gluteal pain is considered to be related to Areas 2 and 3 (Fig. 6.20) [2].

Based on these results, it is more efficient to first inject into Area 0 or 1, in cases with pain from the upper gluteal to groin area, and to inject into Area 2 or 3, in cases with pain in the lower gluteal area [2].

6.1.8 Evaluation of Injection Effect

Postinjection pain was evaluated 15–30 min after the injection in the same manner as the bedside injection, using the pain scale where preinjection pain was set to 10 or by using the visual analogue scale (VAS).

When 70% or more pain was relieved, the injection was judged to be effective. Though most patients felt relief on the same day as their injection, there were some patients whose injections were determined to be effective the following day.

6.1.9 Progress After Injections

Looking at the progress of 27 patients with SIJ-related pain after receiving injections, many patients needed several injections to decrease their pain. However, it

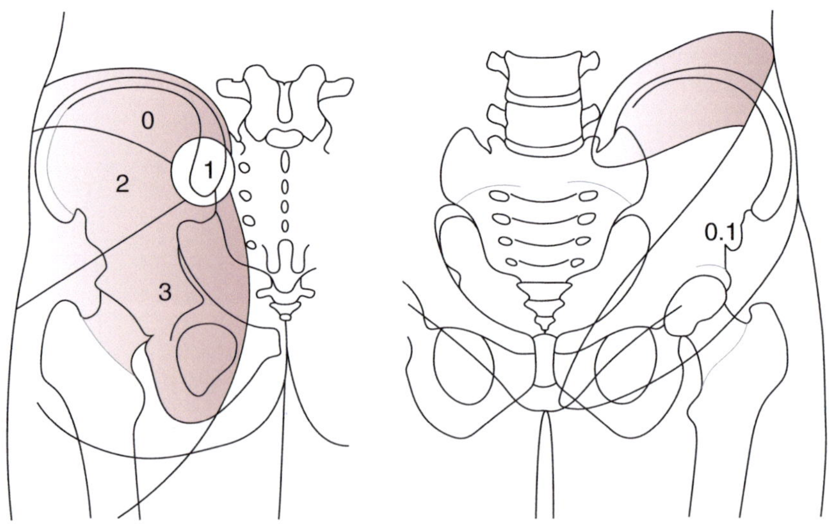

Fig. 6.20 The diagram of the referred pain areas from the four sections. With permission from [7]

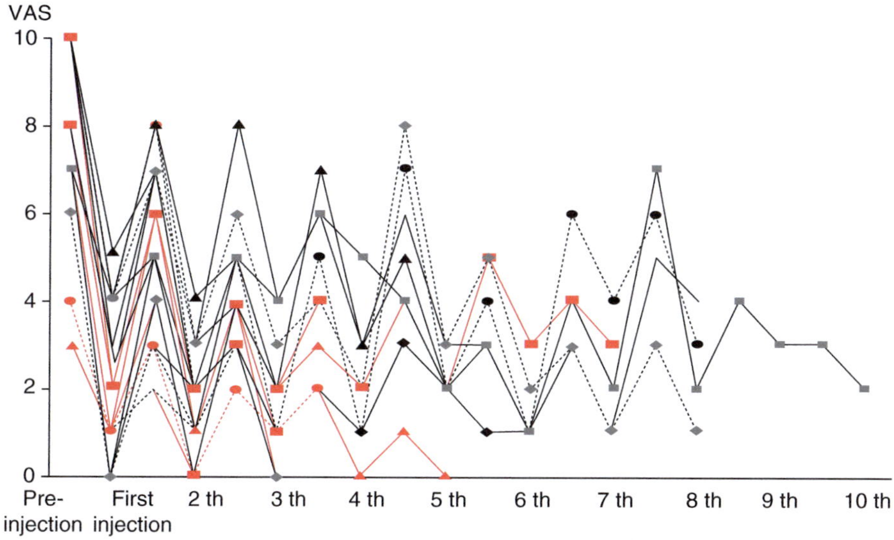

Fig. 6.21 Progress after injections under fluoroscopy. Approximately 80% of the 27 patients had pain relief after several injections (Provided by Daijiro Morimoto, Department of Neurosurgery, Kushiro Rosai Hospital). With permission from [7]

was found that in about 20% of patients, pain was not significantly improved (Fig. 6.21). For those whose injections were not sufficiently effective, treatment methods other than injections were necessary.

6.2 The Peri-Articular Bedside Injection (Fig. 6.22)

The bedside injection is a simple and very useful method that can be done in an outpatient examination room and can obtain a therapeutic effect, though it is less accurate than a fluoroscopic injection.

6.2.1 Comparison of the Positions for an Injection

Best position: slightly bent forward standing position > slightly bent forward sitting position > prone position.

6.2.1.1 The Prone Position

At first, the patient was placed in a prone position (Fig. 6.23a). But in this position, it is not easy to insert a needle cranially from the PSIS to the lower sacrum, because lumbar lordosis usually remains.

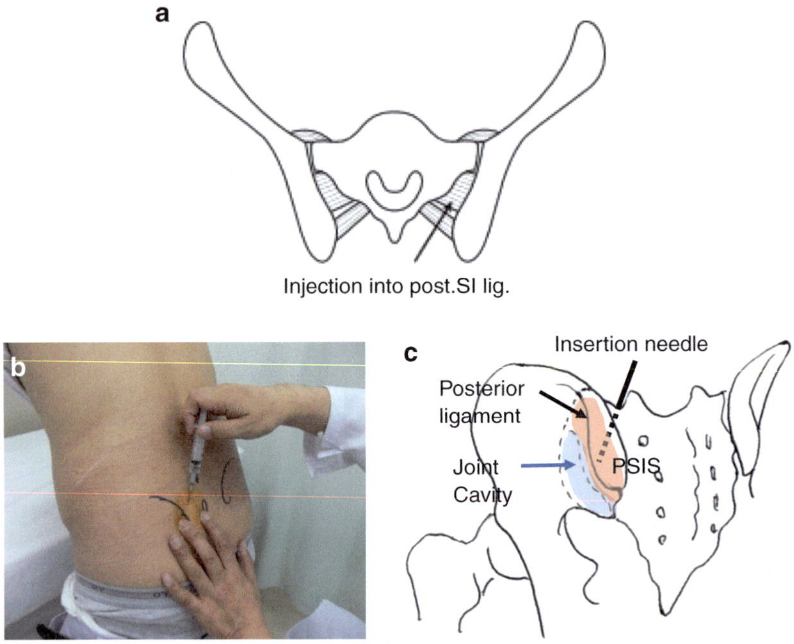

Fig. 6.22 A peri-articular bedside injection. A bedside injection is very easy and suitable for primary care (**a**) the area to be injected. (**b**) an injection scene. (**c**) the direction of an insertion needle

6.2.1.2 The Slightly Bent Forward Standing Position

Currently, the injection is performed with a patient standing about 30–45° bent forward (Fig. 6.23b). By bending forward, a space occurs between the PSIS and the lower lumbar vertebrae, so inserting the needle is made easier.

In addition, when the practitioner sits on a chair, the site for insertion comes near to the eyes of the practitioner. Thus, it becomes easier to insert the needle (Fig. 6.24).

Of course, injection method under ultrasonic guidance is performed to a patient with prone position.

6.2.1.3 The Slightly Bent Forward Sitting Position

In some hospitals, patients are given the injection in a bent forward sitting position while on a chair (Fig. 6.25). As sitting on a chair fixes the iliac bones, the space between the iliac and lumbar spine opens easily when bending forward. However, many patients with SIJ pain have difficulty sitting on chairs, and the site where a needle is inserted while sitting tends to be considerably below the eyeline of the practitioner, and this may make the injection more difficult.

Based on these conditions, we have concluded that the easy position for this procedure is the slightly bent forward standing position.

However, when performing an injection immediately following the examination in the prone position, or when performing an injection under ultrasound guidance,

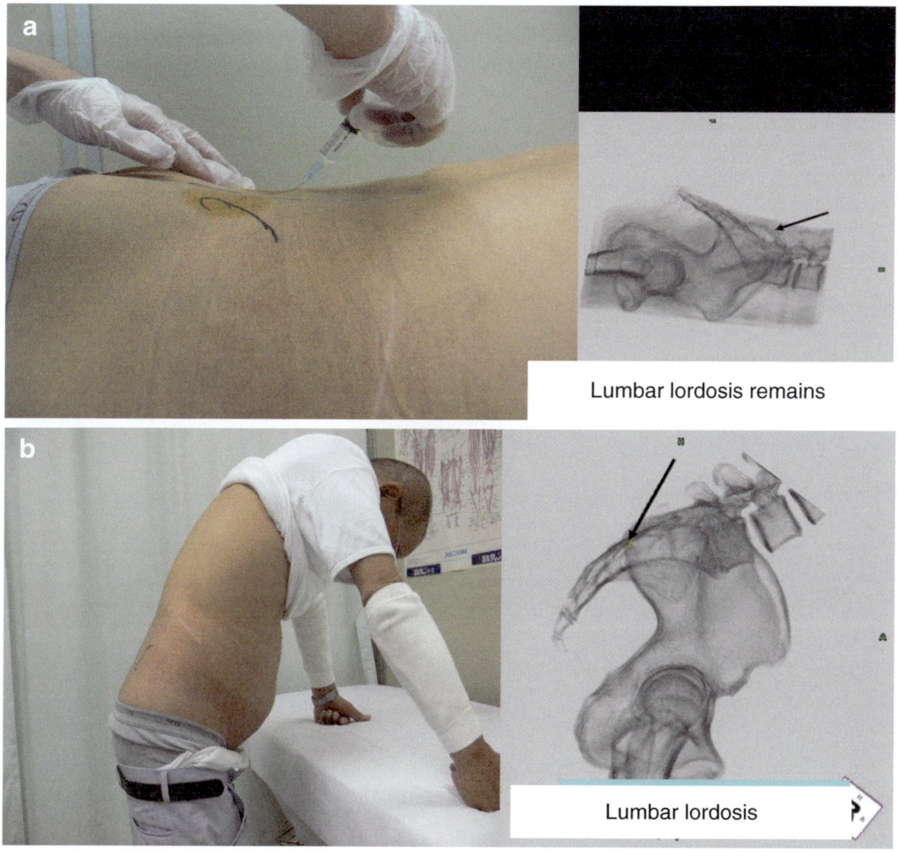

Fig. 6.23 (**a**) An injection in the prone position. In the prone position, it is not easy to insert a needle toward the caudal side since lumbar lordosis remains. (**b**) An injection in the slightly bent forward standing position. This position decreases the lumbar lordosis, so this makes needle insertion easier. With permission from [7]

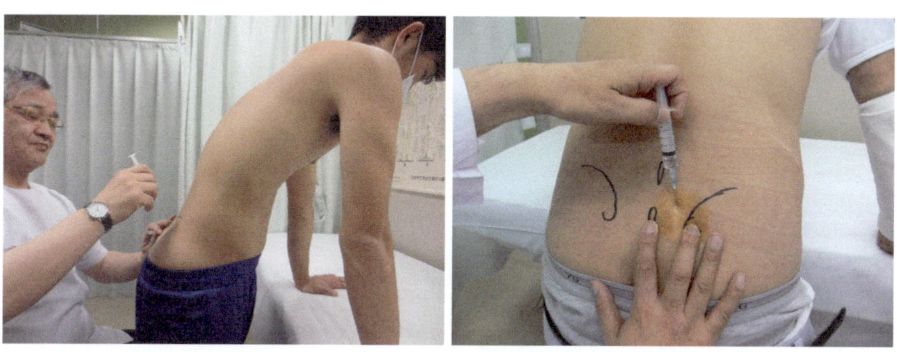

Fig. 6.24 The slightly bent forward standing position makes the insertion become easier, as the insertion site for the needle is nearer to the eyes of the practitioner sitting on a chair

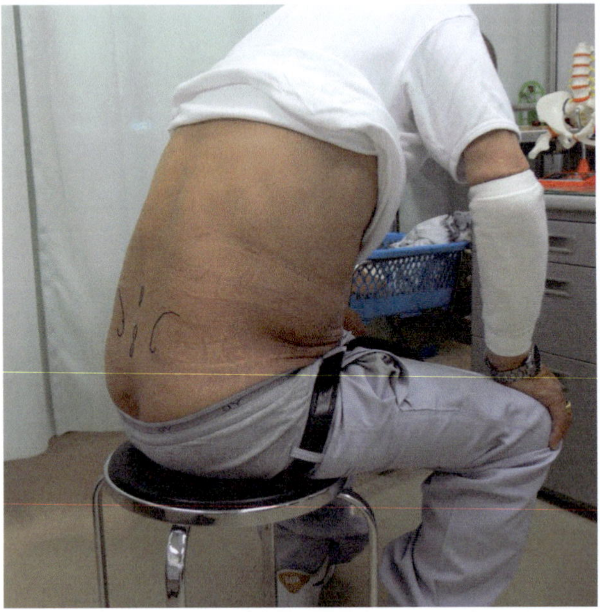

Fig. 6.25 The slightly bent forward sitting position. An injection in the slightly bent forward sitting position is also a good procedure. However, the practitioner needs to insert a needle far below eye level. With permission from [7]

the prone position may be more efficient and better than the bent forward sitting position or standing position.

6.2.2 Items Used for the Bedside Injection (Fig. 6.26)

6.2.2.1 Local Anesthetic Drugs

1% lidocaine (Xylocaine®) is usually used. However, as there have been reports of a few patients who have suffered from anaphylactic shock using lidocaine, some facilities use mepivacaine (Carbocaine®) which is considered to cause anaphylactic shock much less frequently than lidocaine.

6.2.2.2 An Insertion Needle

We usually use a 60-mm 23-gauge needle. We choose the size of the needle based on the strength of the shaft of the needle and of the severity of pain when inserted.

6.2.2.3 An Injection Syringe

We prefer to use a syringe of 5 ml in size. The reason is that a 5 ml syringe is easier to hold like a pen and more sensitive for feeling resistance during an injection of local anesthetic when compared to a 10 ml syringe.

6.2.3 Identification of the PSIS

An indicator for the injection site is the PSIS. The PSIS is a bulge at the posterior, lower end of the ilium. The shape of the PSIS varies from person to person. Moreover, there is difficulty in locating the PSIS on some obese patients.

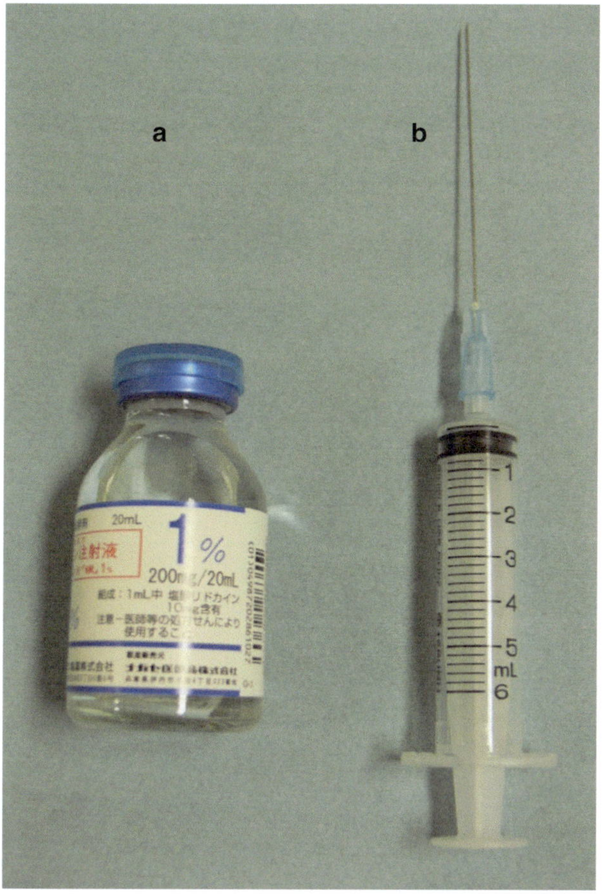

Fig. 6.26 Items for a bedside injection. (**a**) 1% lidocaine (Xylocaine®), (**b**) a 5 ml syringe with a 60-mm 23-gauge needle. With permission from [7]

The identification method of the PSIS is shown below.

6.2.3.1 Identification Method I: Palpating Along the Iliac Crest (Fig. 6.27)

This is a method of touching along the contour of the iliac crest at the low back and tracing from medially to inferiorly along the ilium and reaching the PSIS at the lower end of the iliac crest.

6.2.3.2 Identification Method II: Measuring the PSIS on an X-ray Image (Fig. 6.28)

The distance (a) from the center of the sacrum to the PSIS and the distance (b) between the Jacoby line, which connects the apexes of the left and the right iliac crest, and the PSIS, are measured on an X-ray image of the lower back.

6.2.3.3 Identification Method III: Speculation on CT Measurements (Fig. 6.29)

Using ten cases of Japanese males (height 160–170 cm) and ten cases of Japanese females (height 145–160 cm), we measured the distance (1) from the center of the

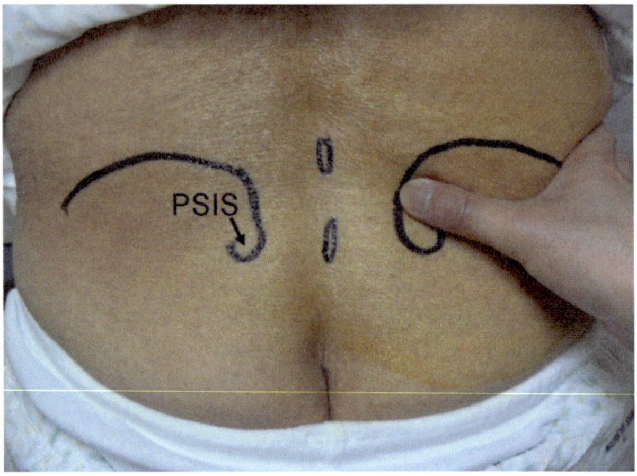

Fig. 6.27 Identification method I of the PSIS. While touching the iliac crest with your finger and tracing the bone medially, identify the PSIS at the posterior lower end of the iliac bone. With permission from [7]

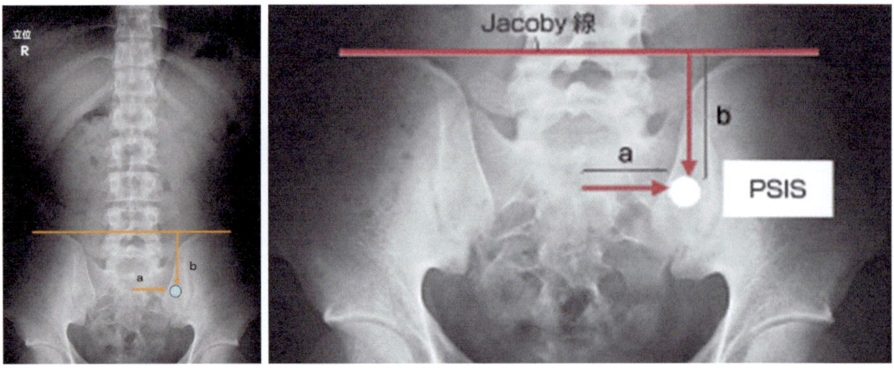

Fig. 6.28 Identification method II of the PSIS. Based on the distances measured on an X-ray image of the lower back (*a*: the distance from the center of the sacrum to the PSIS, *b*: the distance between the Jacoby line and the PSIS). The PSIS can be identified on the patient. With permission from [7]

sacrum to the PSIS and the distance (2) from the line connecting the apexes of both the left and right iliac crests to the PSIS. Based on these measurements, the averages for (1) and (2) are 44 ± 5.2 mm and 55 ± 5.6 mm for males and 48 ± 4.4 mm and 47 ± 7.3 mm for females, respectively. Based on these data, the site of the PSIS can be speculated.

6.2.4 The Direction for Needle Insertion

A needle is inserted into the ligamentous region between the sacrum and the ilium. The central compartment (Area 2) among the four sections in the posterior area of the SIJ has the highest rate of reproducing familiar pain [1] (Table 6.1). Hence, you should aim for Area 2 first and aim for Area 3, which is the lower

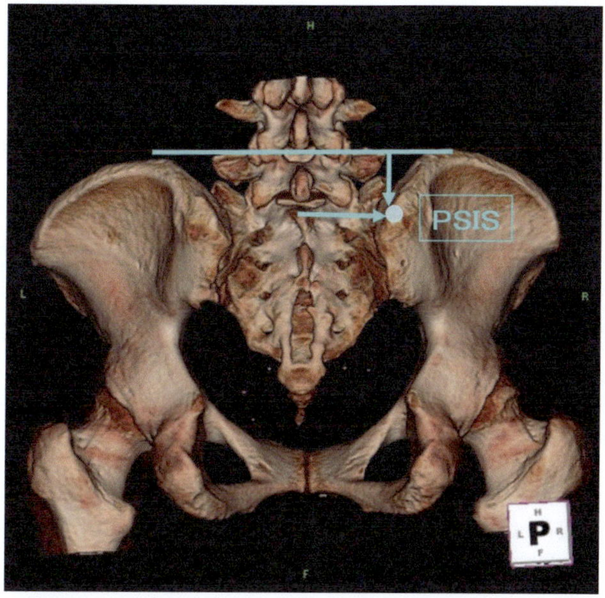

Fig. 6.29 Identification method III of the PSIS. Identify the PSIS by referring to an averaged distance obtained from CT images of ten male and female individuals (Japanese) (1: from the center of the sacrum to the PSIS, 2: from the line (Jacoby line) connecting the apexes of the left and right iliac crests to the PSIS). With permission from [7]

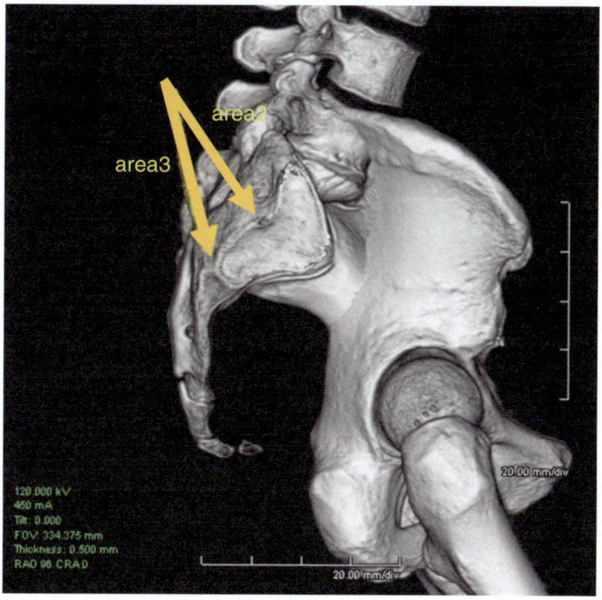

Fig. 6.30 Initially the needle insertion aiming for Area 2 and Area 3 should be efficient. With permission from [7]

posterior area of the SIJ, next (Fig. 6.30). For efficient needle insertion, aim at the medial border of the PSIS. In order to allow the needle to directly reach the ligamentous region behind the SIJ, it is best to insert the needle into the medial border of the PSIS.

6.2.4.1 The Direction for a Safe Insertion of the Needle: Inserting the Needle from the Cranial Side of the PSIS

If a needle is inserted from the cranial side of the PSIS into the caudal side ((1) in Fig. 6.31), there is little possibility that the needle may penetrate the pelvic cavity. CT image shows that the posterior region of the SIJ is covered with thick ligaments between the sacrum and the ilium and the joint line is curved irregularly. So it is almost impossible that a needle can penetrate through the thick ligaments and the curved joint space, into the pelvic cavity, even if the needle is inserted toward the pelvic cavity (Fig. 6.32). If the needle is inserted more horizontally, it moves away from the pelvic cavity ((2) in Fig. 6.31).

Consequently, if it is inserted from the cranial side of the PSIS, there is no worry of the needle penetrating the pelvic cavity.

On one occasion, I tried to forcefully insert a needle into the joint space through the posterior ligaments of the joint space but could not do it.

6.2.4.2 A Safe and Effective Needle Insertion

Inserting the needle medially from the cranial side of the PSIS toward the lateral caudal side and passing along the inner edge of the PSIS is safe and effective (Fig. 6.33).

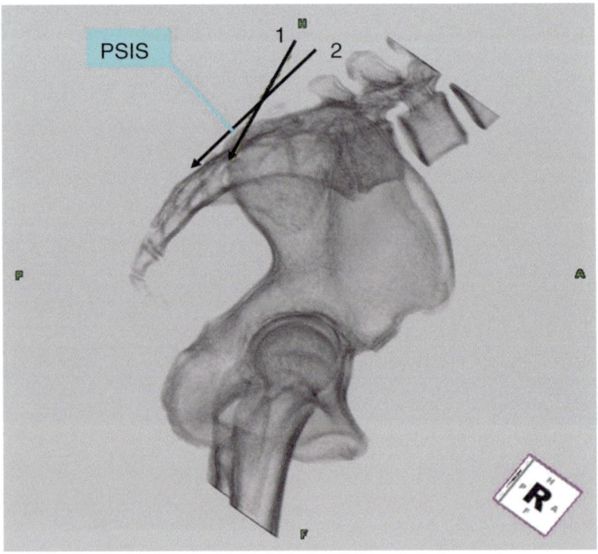

Fig. 6.31 Safe insertion of the needle (=safe needle insertion). Inserting a needle from the cranial side of the PSIS downward (1) is not dangerous. If the needle is inserted more horizontally, it moves away from the pelvic cavity (2). With permission from [7]

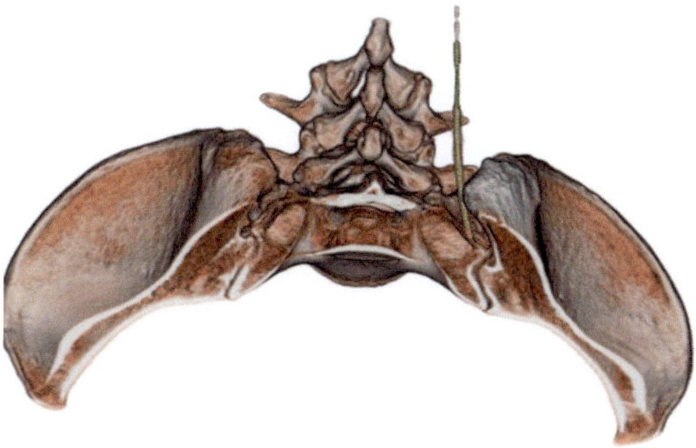

Fig. 6.32 Risk of the needle penetrating the pelvic cavity. It is unlikely that the needle will penetrate the pelvic cavity, a needle insertion from the cranial side of the PSIS because of the thick posterior ligaments and the irregularly curved joint space. With permission from [7]

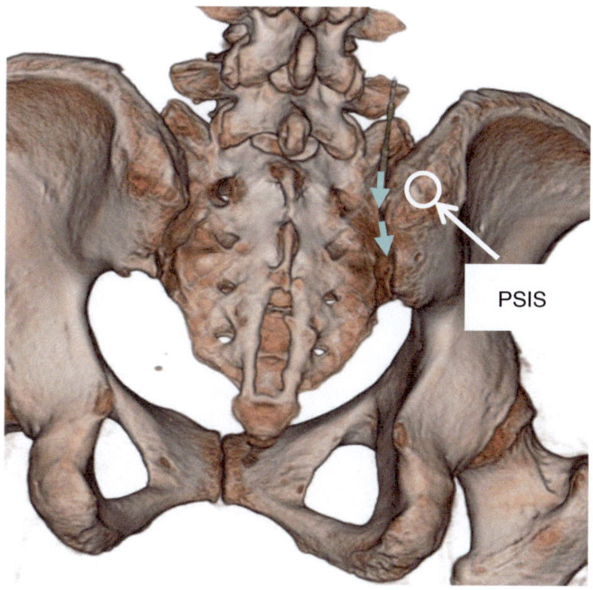

Fig. 6.33 The direction for a safe and effective needle insertion

6.2.5 Actual Procedure of a Needle Insertion

6.2.5.1 The Slightly Bent Forward Standing Position

First, a patient stands facing the examination table and bends forward about 30–45°.

6.2.5.2 Needle Insertion

Using a 60-mm 23-gauge needle

The Insertion Point 1–2 cm medially and 2 cm cranially from the PSIS. The direction of the needle should be slightly lateral toward the caudal side and pass along the inner edge of the PSIS. The needle should be angled ±10° from the vertical axis toward the practitioner or the patient, often being at roughly a right angle to

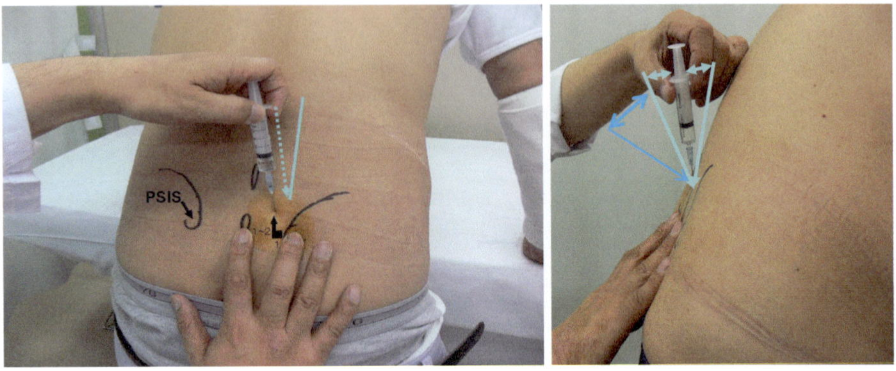

Fig. 6.34 Points of needle insertion. First, a patient stands facing the examination table and bends forward about 30–45°. Using a 60-mm 23-gauge needle. The insertion point: 1~2 cm medially and 2 cm cranially from the PSIS. The direction of insertion: slightly laterally toward the caudal side and passing along the inner edge of the PSIS. The angle of the needle: ±10° from the vertical axis toward the practitioner or patient, often toward right angle to the surface of the back. After inserting the needle, inject 2~3 ml of 1% lidocaine. With permission from [7]

the surface of the back (Fig. 6.34). In this procedure, we can aim near the central compartment (Area 2) of the SIJ. If we angle the needle caudally, we can aim for the caudal compartment (Area 3).

However, *do not be nervous about the angle of the needle!* It is most important to find the area where the familiar pain is induced by a needle insertion.

Furthermore, a needle insertion from a more cranial position is necessary in order to aim for the cranial sections (Areas 0 and 1).

Since the procedure is a blind insertion, it is not possible to exactly confirm where the needle tip may be located. However, by adjusting the direction of the needle, it should be possible to insert a needle into the four sections (0–3) (Fig. 6.35a, b).

6.2.6 Important Points for Bedside Injections

6.2.6.1 Hunting for the Area Where the Familiar Pain Is Induced by a Needle Insertion Is Very Important

If a needle is inserted into the pain origin, familiar pain is induced. No matter how old the patient is, they can feel whether the needle has been inserted near the source of pain. If an inserted needle is separated from the pain origin by only a few mm, the familiar pain is not induced. In some patients, the familiar pain is reproduced during the injection of local anesthetic. When the familiar pain is induced, the injection of local anesthetic is obviously more effective than that without the familiar pain.

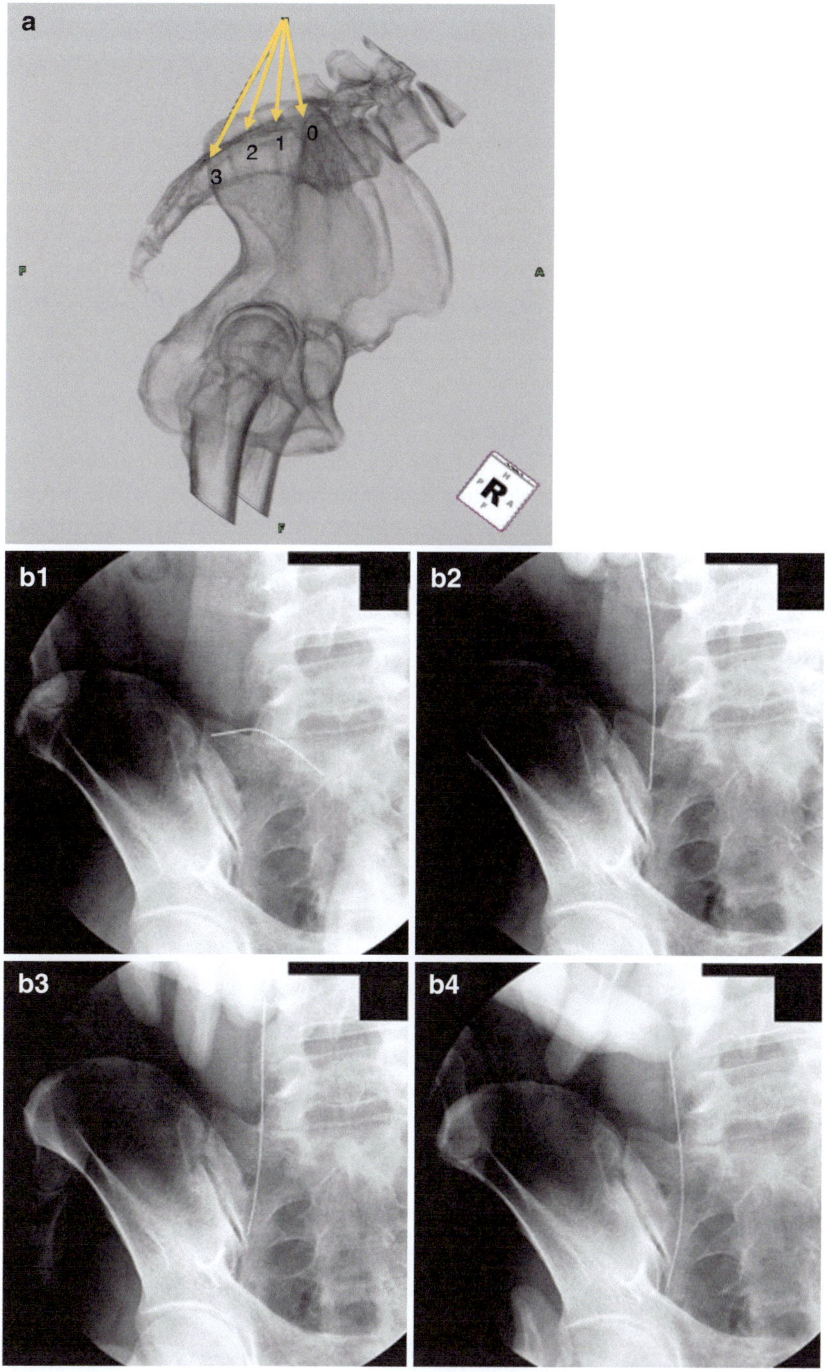

Fig. 6.35 (**a**) A needle insertion into the four sections (0–3) may be possible by adjusting the direction of the needle skillfully. (**b**) X-ray of a needle insertion into the four sections (0–3). (b-1, Area 0; b-2, Area 1; b-3, Area 2; b-4, Area 3) With permission from [7]

Key Message: The Path of the Needle

The path of the needle in a 50-year-old female receiving an SIJ injection (Fig. 6.36).

At the skin penetration point, a needle is inserted medially and cranially from the PSIS (Fig. 6.36a).

It passes through the spinal erector muscles (Fig. 6.36b). As it is inserted deeper, it penetrates the interosseous sacroiliac ligament (Fig. 6.36c). Finally, the needle arrives at the gap between the sacrum and the inner edge of the PSIS (Fig. 6.36d). The oblique view of her CT image shows the needle inserted into the central compartment (Area2) (Fig. 6.36e).

6.2.6.2 When Inserting for Area 0

When aiming for Area 0, you should hit the needle on the sacrum and then insert it in order to avoid the risk of penetrating the abdominal cavity (Fig. 6.37). Since the bedside injection is a blind procedure, you should not repeatedly try insertions into this section. Fluoroscopic injection is safer to perform an insertion, if you do not have confidence to perform it successfully.

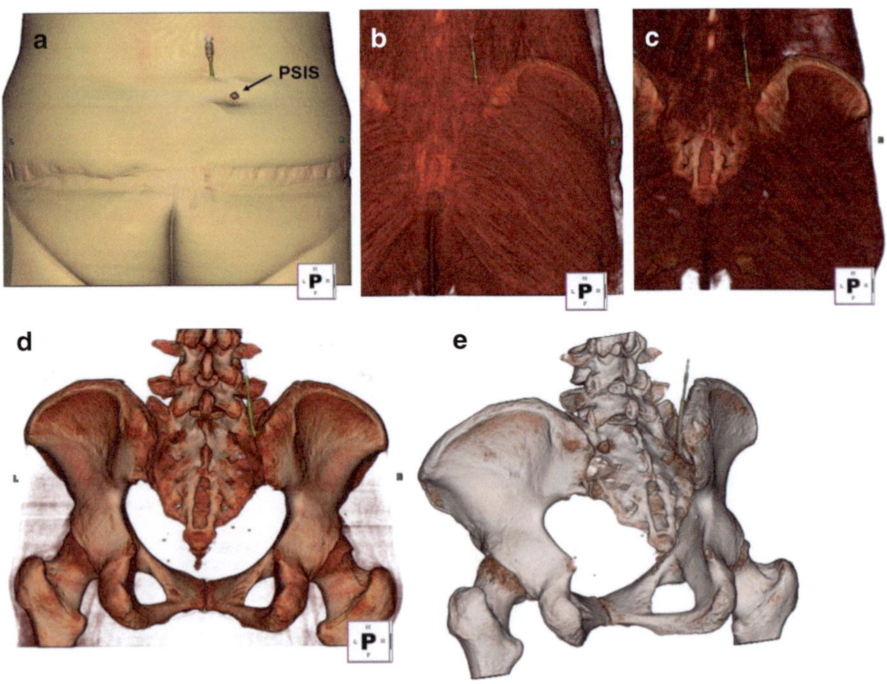

Fig. 6.36 (**a**) The skin penetration point. (**b**) The site of the needle penetrating muscle. (**c**) The site of insertion into the interosseous sacroiliac ligament. (**d**) AP view on CT of the insertion into the gap between the sacrum and the inner edge of the PSIS. (**e**) The oblique view on CT. With permission from [7]

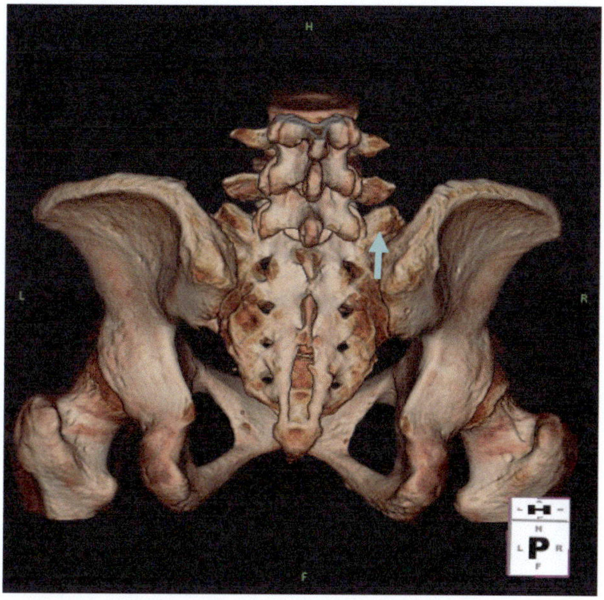

Fig. 6.37 When aiming for Area 0, inserting the needle after hitting it on the sacrum is necessary

6.2.6.3 Limits and Risks of an Injection from the Caudal Side of the PSIS

Some people insert the injection needle from below the PSIS.

However, when using this approach, aiming for Areas 0 and 1 is difficult, owing to the PSIS acting as a barrier (white arrow). Furthermore, there is also the possibility that the needle may be inserted into the pelvic cavity (red arrow) (Fig. 6.38).

6.2.7 When a Needle Becomes Obstructed

6.2.7.1 The Cause for the Needle Not Advancing

Often the needle strikes the inner edge of the PSIS (Fig. 6.39).

It is important to have the needle pass along the inner edge of the PSIS skillfully.

6.2.7.2 Techniques for Advancing the Needle

One technique is rotating the needle. When doing so, the tip of the needle sometimes slips and can be smoothly inserted (Fig. 6.40a).

When the needle still cannot be advanced, it should be inserted more caudally (Fig. 6.40b) or more horizontally to the skin (Fig. 6.40c).

When you cannot advance it by any means, move the insertion point more inward and perform the injection again (Fig. 6.40d).

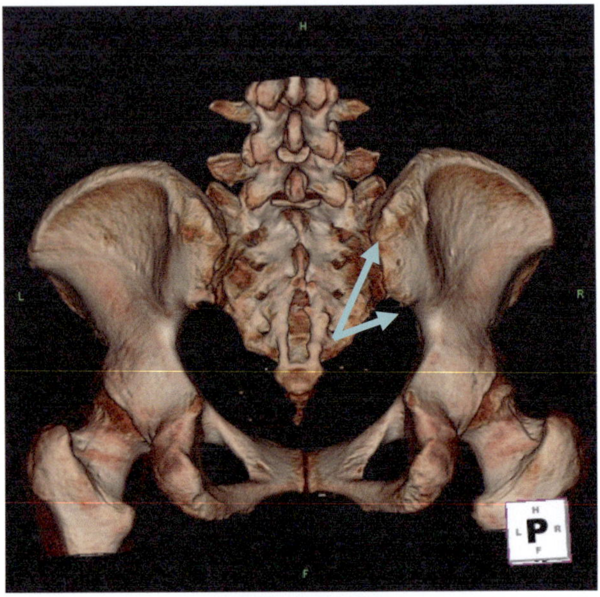

Fig. 6.38 An injection from the caudal side of the PSIS. With permission from [7]

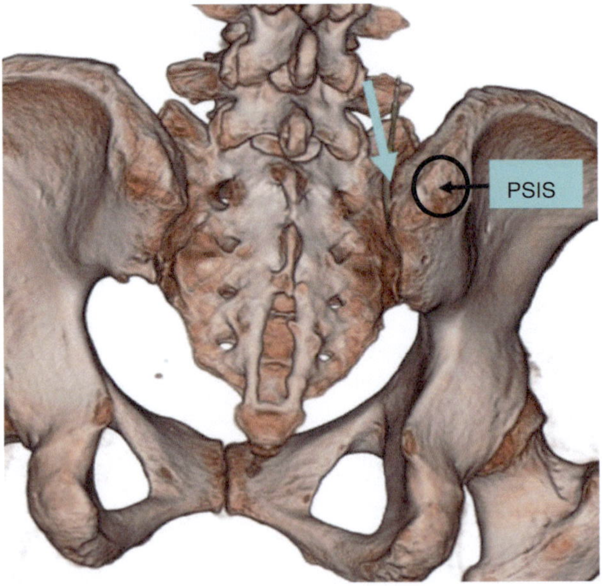

Fig. 6.39 The cause for the needle not advancing. The needle is often obstructed by the inner edge of the PSIS. With permission from [7]

6.2.8 The Depth of the Needle, Injection Dose of Local Anesthetic Used, Infusion Speed, and Evaluation After an Injection

6.2.8.1 The Depth of the Needle

Do not be nervous about the depth of the needle.

When a needle reaches the pain origin, most patients can feel the familiar pain and may say something like "this is my pain." It is enough only to inject a local anesthetic at the depth where the familiar pain is reproduced. However, for the

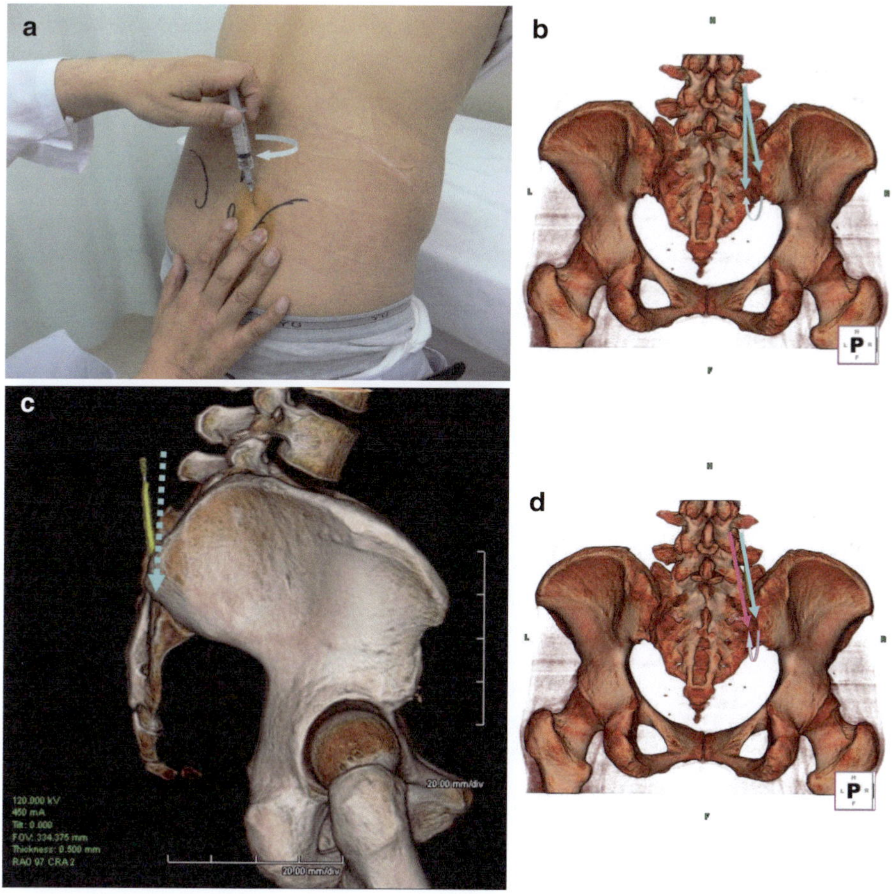

Fig. 6.40 Techniques for advancing the needle. (**a**) When rotating the needle, the tip of the needle sometimes slips and can be smoothly inserted. (**b**) Insert the needle more caudally (white arrow). (**c**) If the needle hit the sacrum, angle it more horizontally to the skin and insert it. (**d**) If the needle does not advance by any means, move the insertion point more inward and reinsert the needle (white arrow). With permission from [7]

bedside injection, it is more important to find the area where the familiar pain is induced by a needle insertion than by relying on the depth of the needle.

If the practitioner feels the needle penetrate ligaments or reach deep bone, and the patient says "this is my pain" when inserting the needle or injecting a small amount of local anesthetic, the injection should be effective (Fig. 6.41).

6.2.8.2 Injection Dose of Local Anesthetic

For the injection dose of local anesthetic: 2–3 ml of local anesthetic is sufficient for injection into the area where patient's familiar pain is reproduced.

Any more than the above dose may cause the anesthetic to spread into other areas. We have had some patients who had temporary numbness and weakness of the affected lower limb immediately after an injection. It is considered that the local anesthetic injected probably spread into the sciatic nerve.

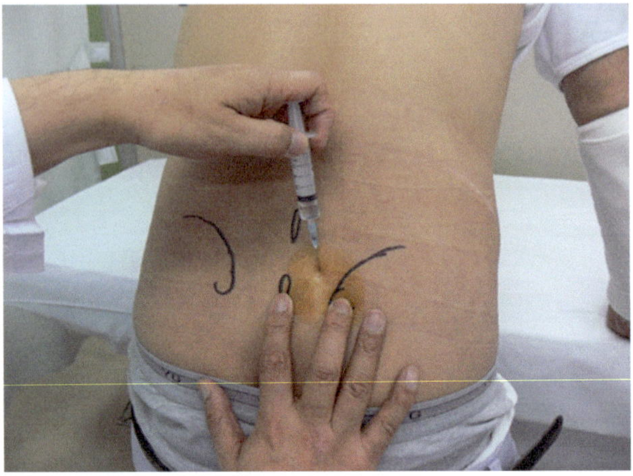

Fig. 6.41 Optimal depth of the needle for the injection of local anesthetic. The injection is effective at the depth where the patient says "this is my pain." It is important to find the area where the familiar pain is reproduced by inserting a needle or by injecting a small amount of local anesthetic. With permission from [7]

6.2.8.3 Infusion Speed for Local Anesthetic: A Forceful Injection is Dangerous

Since the area to receive the local anesthetic is a narrow space covered with thick ligaments, be very careful of the infusion speed. When there is severe resistance, you must not inject the local anesthetic forcefully.

I have encountered some patients having intense pain, lasting for several days, after forcing an injection of local anesthetic despite feeling hard resistance. When there is severe resistance, it is important to lower the infusion speed or slightly withdraw the needle and inject the local anesthetic at a site with less resistance.

6.2.8.4 Evaluation of Injection Effectiveness

Postinjection pain was evaluated 15–30 min after the injection using the pain scale where preinjection pain was set to 10 or by using the visual analogue scale (VAS).

Key Message: Injection Method Under Ultrasonic Guidance

These days, an injection method using an ultrasonic device has come to be popular (Fig. 6.42a). The ultrasonic device can clearly show the gap between the inner edge of the PSIS and the sacrum. This facilitates the insertion of the needle (Fig. 6.42b).

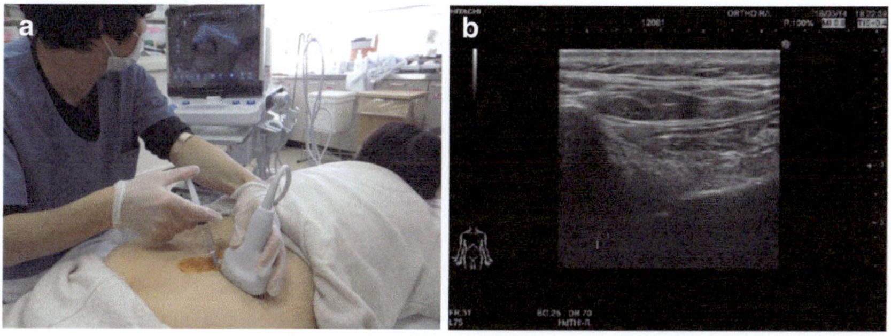

Fig. 6.42 Ultrasound-guided injection method. (**a**) Injection using an ultrasonic device. (**b**) The gap between the inner edge of the PSIS and the sacrum can be confirmed

6.2.9 Summary of the Procedure for Bedside Injections (Fig. 6.43)

6.2.9.1 Positioning of the Patient

The patient stands facing the examination table and bends forward about 30–45°.

6.2.9.2 Identification of the PSIS

The methods for identifying the PSIS mentioned above are useful.

6.2.9.3 Insertion of the Needle

The practitioner puts his/her index finger and middle finger on the PSIS and the center of the sacrum, respectively. The practitioner holds a 5 ml syringe with a 60-mm 23-gauge needle like a pen in the other hand. 1–2 cm medially and 2 cm cranially from the PSIS, the needle is inserted slightly laterally toward the caudal side and passes along the inner edge of the PSIS.

6.2.9.4 Injection of Local Anesthetic

While feeling the needle penetrates the ligaments or strikes the sacrum, at a depth where the patient says "right there" or "this is my pain," gently inject 2–3 ml of local anesthetic after confirming that the blood has not been sucked into the barrel of the syringe.

6.2.9.5 Evaluation After the Injection

At 15–30 min after the injection, the effect of the injection is evaluated using the pain scale or the visual analogue scale. If pain relief is evaluated at 50% or more, the bedside injection has been effective.

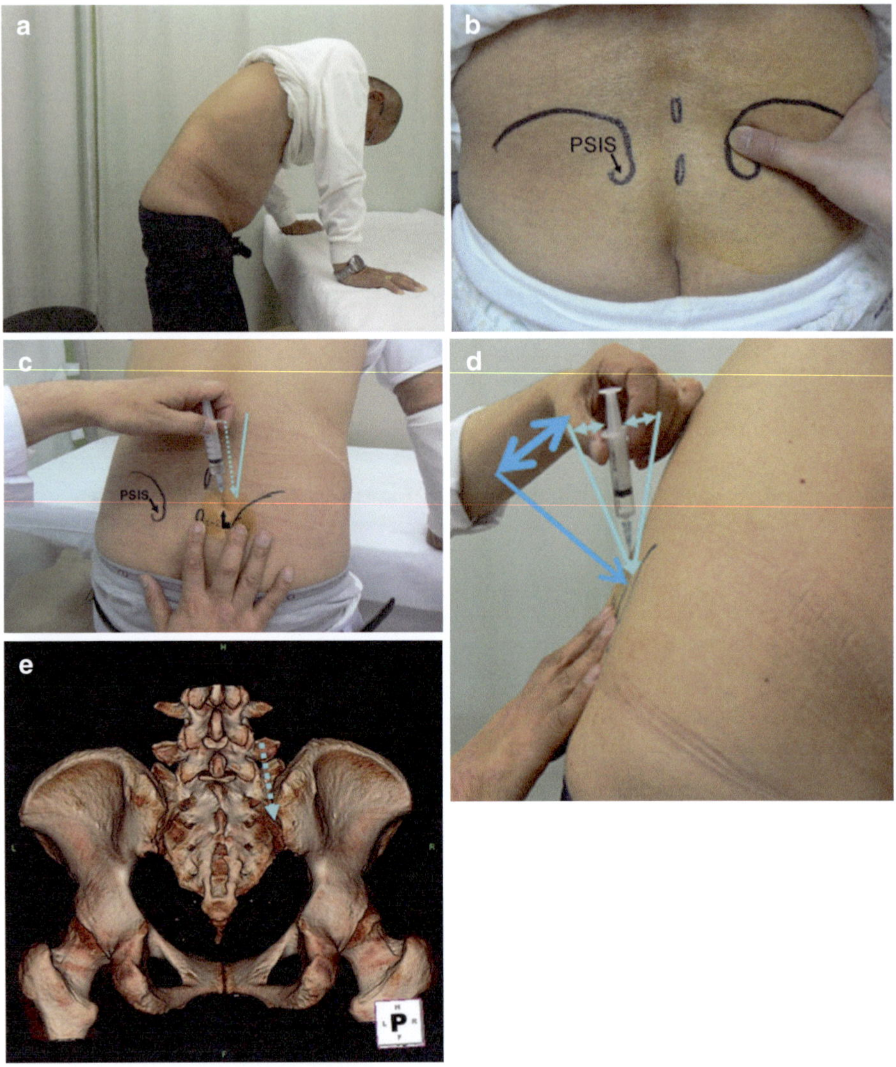

Fig. 6.43 The procedure for bedside injection. (**a**) A patient stands bent forward about 30–45°. (**b**) Identification of the PSIS. (**c**) Insertion of the needle. Putting the practitioner's fingers on the PSIS and the center of the sacrum, respectively. 1–2 cm medially and 2 cm cranially from the PSIS, the needle is inserted slightly laterally toward the caudal side. (**d**) The needle is inserted at an angle of ±10° from the vertical axis toward the practitioner. Often toward right angle to surface of the back. (**e**) Passing along the inner edge of the PSIS. With permission from [7]

Key Message: The Path to Instantly Recognize SIJ Pain

If a needle for a trigger point injection to the low back area is adjusted caudally and reinserted from a more caudal point, it should reach the posterior SI ligament. We would instantly recognize the patient suffers from SIJ pain when seeing the pain dramatically relieved after the injection (Fig. 6.44).

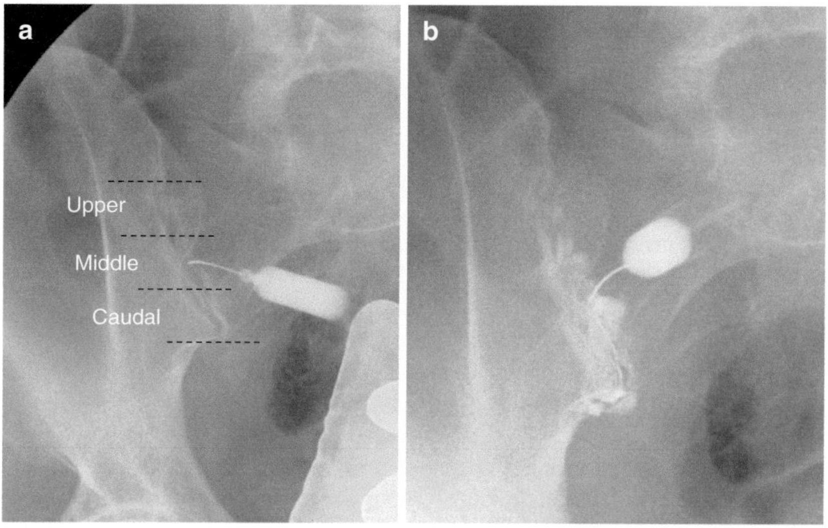

Fig. 6.44 A new intra-articular SIJ injection via the middle portion of the joint. (**a**) Needle insertion via the middle portion of the joint. (**b**) Intra-articular arthrogram

6.3 The Intra-Articular Injection

Kurosawa's technique is recommended [3].

Several previous studies have reported that it is often not possible to gain access into the SIJ [4–6]; clinically, successful intra-articular injection is not easy. If an intra-articular injection is needed, Kurosawa's technique [3] is recommended because his personal success rate was higher, as much as 80%, and easier to perform than the conventional technique described by the previous studies (Fig. 6.44).

6.3.1 Supplies/Necessary Items for an Injection (Fig. 6.45a)

Like a peri-articular injection:

Insertion needle: A 90-mm 23-gauge spinal needle (or a 60-mm 23-gauge needle) is used on occasion.

A syringe: A 2.5 ml syringe for more minute injection.

The local anesthetic: We usually use 2% lidocaine for the local anesthetic and a steroid because patients with effective intra-articular injection would have inflammation in the cavity. In order to confirm the needle's entry into the joint cavity, a contrast medium in a 2.5 ml syringe is used first. After outlining the joint, the local anesthetic is injected.

6.3.2 Procedure

With the patient lying prone-oblique with the painful side down on a fluoroscopy table, the posterior SIJ line is divided into four sections, as shown in our previous studies according to the peri-articular injection technique. A 90-mm 23-gauge spinal needle was inserted into the middle portion of the joint, which was designated as Area 2 in our previous study (Fig. 6.45b).

A needle is inserted into the point where the joint line intersects with the parallel lines formed by the inferior border of the PSIS and the border of the lateral sacral crest. The needle is advanced nearly perpendicular to the fluoroscopic beam. After the needle has been inserted and advanced to the bone, the fluoroscopy tube is angled caudally 25–30°. With this technique, the image clearly shows the recess between the ilium and the sacrum (Fig. 6.46).

The needle direction should be adjusted under fluoroscopic guidance to the clearly detectable posterior margin of the joint. When the needle has been advanced until it has reached the bone wall of the ilium in the middle portion, contrast medium is injected (Fig. 6.47).

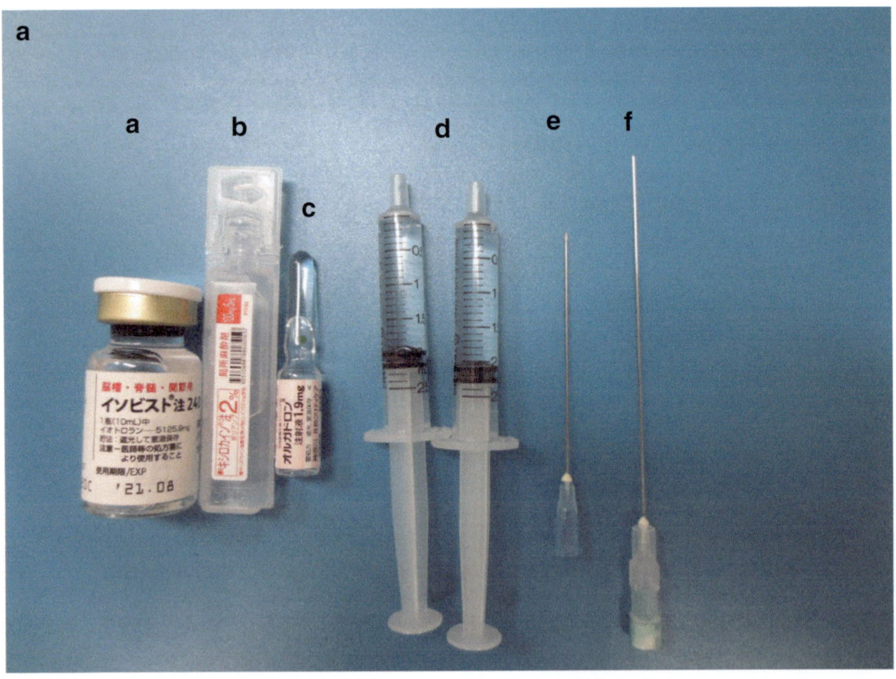

Fig. 6.45 (**a**) Items for an intra-articular injection. *a*: Omnipark® 240 (contrast medium), *b*: 2% lidocaine, *c*: steroid drug, *d*: 2.5 ml syringe, *e*: a 60-mm 23-G needle, *f*: a 90-mm 23-G spinal needle. (**b**) The approach via the middle portion of the joint. An entry point of a needle is the middle portion of the joint which is into Area 2 in the peri-articular region

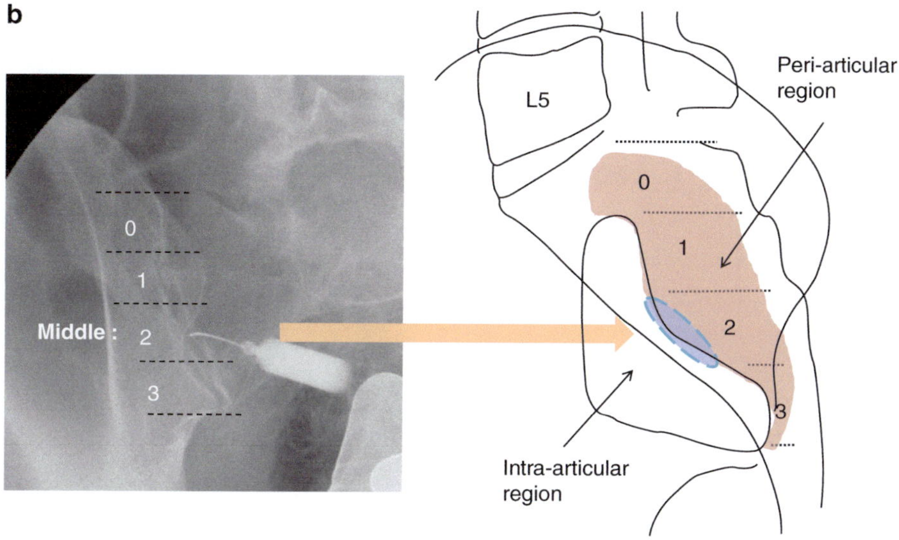

Fig. 6.45 (continued)

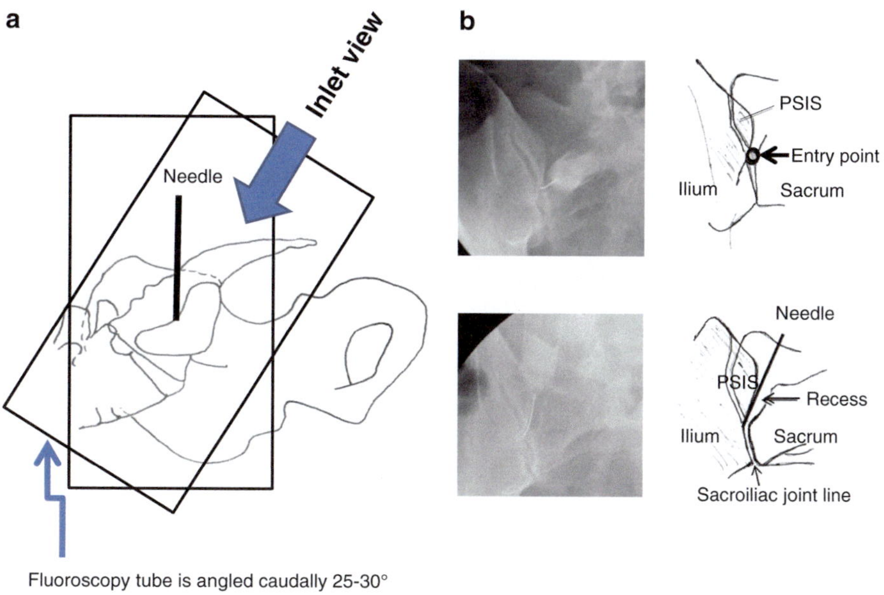

Fig. 6.46 Technical procedure 1. (**a**) A needle is inserted at an entry point (into Area 2) where the joint line intersects with the inferior border of the PSIS and the border of the lateral sacral crest. (**b**) After needle insertion, a fluoroscopic image angled caudally 25–30°. The inlet view allows us to check the needle direction and depth in the recess between the ilium and the sacrum [3]

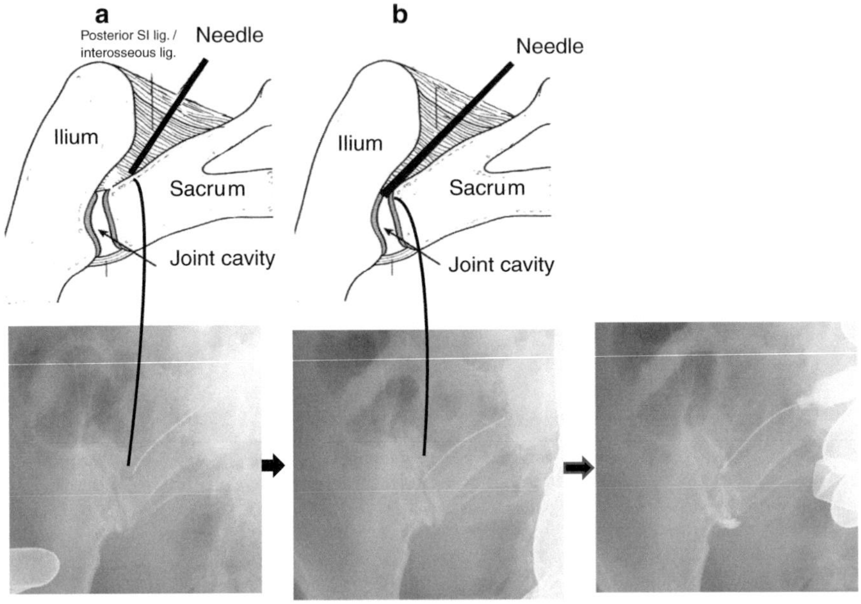

Fig. 6.47 Technical procedure 2. (**a**) The needle is advanced while adjusting its direction to the posterior margin of the joint. (**b**) When the needle reaches the ilium, contrast medium is injected. Adapted from A. Vleeming et al. (Eds.). Movement, Stability and Lumbopelvic Pain 2nd Edition. 2007 [8]

When the tip of the needle reaches the cartilage, it could be felt by your finger through the needle. Usually the needle can access the joint cavity without obstruction by the dense ligaments in the middle portion. After outlining the joint, 1.5–2.0 ml of 2% lidocaine is injected. If the contrast medium leaks on the first attempt, you should change the needle direction slightly. It can be confirmed that the local anesthetic has been injected into joint cavity correctly by a whole shadow of the contrast medium diffused in the joint.

If the needle cannot reach the posterior margin of the joint, a contra-oblique view technique will help the needle to be inserted into the joint cavity (Fig. 6.48).

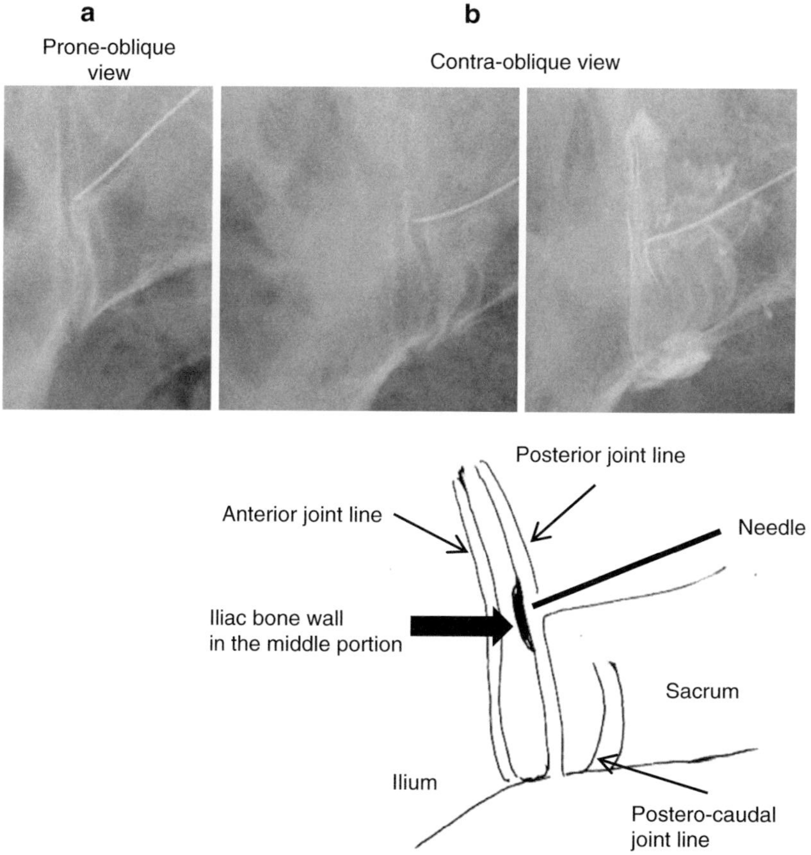

Fig. 6.48 Contra-oblique view technique. (**a**) When the needle cannot reach the posterior margin of the joint in prone-oblique with the painful side down. (**b**) Rotating the patient in a contra-oblique direction. When the needle tip has accessed to the ilium beyond the border of the sacrum, it should be inserted into the joint cavity. A contra-oblique view will show whether the needle tip should be situated inside the posterior joint line [3]

References

1. Murakami E, Tanaka Y, Aizawa T, et al. Effect of periarticular and intraarticular lidocaine injections for sacroiliac joint pain: a prospective comparative study. J Orthop Sci. 2007;12:274–80.
2. Kurosawa D, Murakami E, Aizawa T. Referred pain location depends on the affected section of the sacroiliac joint. Eur Spine J. 2015;24:521–7.
3. Kurosawa D, Murakami E, Aizawa T. Fluoroscopy-guided sacroiliac intraarticular injection via the middle portion of the joint: a technical report. Pain Med. 2017;18:1642.
4. Hendrix RW, Lin PP, Kane WJ. Simplified aspiration of injection technique for the sacroiliac joint. J Bone Joint Surg Am. 1982;64:1249–52.
5. Dussault RG, Kaplan PA, Anderson MW. Fluoroscopy-guided sacroiliac joint injections. Radiology. 2000;214:273–7.

6. Gupta S. Double needle technique: an alternative method for performing difficult sacroiliac joint injections. Pain Physician. 2011;14:281–4.
7. Murakami E. Sacroiliac joint pain: undiagnosed low back pain. Tokyo: Nankodo; 2012. (in Japanese).
8. Vleeming A, Mooney V, Stoeckart R. Movement, stability & lumbopelvic pain: integration of research and therapy. 2nd ed. Edinburgh: Elsevier; 2007.

Improvements and Prevention of Sacroiliac Joint Disorder

7

Abstract

- A rubber pelvic belt and an exercise ball are useful items to improve SIJ disorder.
- Points for preventing SIJ disorder include not working in the same posture for a long time and active walking. Do not be relaxed while in semi-flexion posture or during activity.
- The transversus abdominis muscle and gluteus maximus muscle are important in stabilizing the SIJ.
- The draw-in exercise and the bridge exercise are effective in training the transversus abdominis and the gluteus maximus.
- Squatting exercise is effective for maintaining the function of the SIJ.

7.1 Differences in the Pelvis of Males and Females [1]

The pelvic ring consists of two pelvic bones and a sacrum with the SIJs at the posterior and the pubic syndesmosis at the anterior.

It constitutes the base of the trunk and supports the abdomen, as well. The pelvic ring connects the spinal column to the lower extremities. The pelvis resembles a funnel which is wider at the top. The shape of the pelvis differs between men and women. The female pelvis has a wider opening at the base of the pelvis than the male pelvis. Conversely, the height of the female pelvis has been detected to be shorter than the male pelvis. In addition, the female pelvis opens widely at the top and forms a structure which can allow the head of a baby to easily pass through during delivery (Fig. 7.1).

E. Murakami, *Sacroiliac Joint Disorder*,
https://doi.org/10.1007/978-981-13-1807-8_7

7.2 Useful Items to Improve SIJ Disorder

7.2.1 A Rubber Pelvic Belt (see Fig. 5.6)

You can expect sufficient pain relief by having the patient put on a pelvic belt below the iliac crest.

7.2.2 An Exercise Ball (Fig. 7.2)

An exercise ball is thought to promote an automatic reaction which is necessary to the functioning of the SIJ [2]. Movement on an exercise ball can be effective for strengthening the inner muscles, such as the abdominal transverse muscle, because it requires cooperative movement and proper reflex of the inner muscle groups in order to maintain vertical stability.

Key Message: Utility of an Exercise Ball (Fig. 7.2)
I realized the true effectiveness of an exercise ball when I treated a female patient with SIJ disorder.

Even when SIJ injections were repeated, the effectiveness of them would not last.

I was in trouble because I was at a loss for another practical treatment. However, one day the patient suddenly said "I got better."

When I asked her what kind of treatment she had undergone, she said that her pain had been relieved after alternately raising both legs while on an exercise ball.

Since then, the woman has continued using the exercise ball and her symptoms have improved over time.

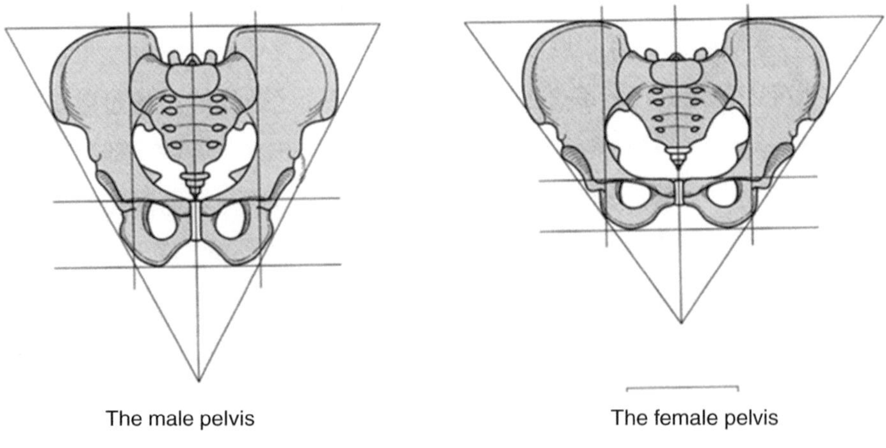

Fig. 7.1 Differences of the pelvis in males and females. The male pelvis is slightly narrower than the female pelvis. Women have a wider and shorter pelvic cavity than men (Kapandji IA (Author), Hagijima Hideo (Translation): Physiology of the Kapandi Joint III, Trunk and Spine, Medical Toothpaste Ed., Tokyo, p. 49, 1986). With permission from [8]

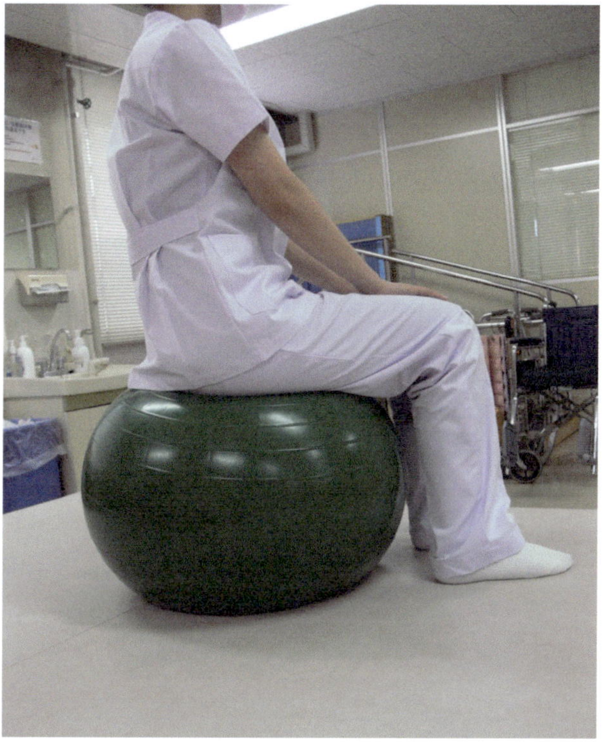

Fig. 7.2 An exercise ball. Movement on an exercise ball can be effective for strengthening the inner muscles and promoting an automatic reaction of the muscles. With permission from [8]

7.3 Prevention of SIJ Disorder

7.3.1 Points for Preventing SIJ Disorder (Fig. 7.3)

7.3.1.1 Avoid Working in the Same Posture for a Long Time

Muscles around the low back and pelvis, whether sitting or standing, are forced to act. Therefore, if you keep the same posture, such as when driving a car or sitting, the cooperative action of muscles around the SIJs is reduced due to muscle fatigue, and joint dysfunction tends to occur. In order to prevent this, it is effective to interrupt work roughly every 30 min and perform the extension and flexion of the lumbar spine and the rolling of the hip and waist.

7.3.1.2 Do Not Be Relaxed While in Semi-flexion Posture or During Action

In the SIJ, it is said that a semi-flexed posture is in the most loosely packed position. Therefore, when holding objects or washing the face in this posture, be careful because minor subluxation or catching of the joints is likely to occur. Injury of the lumbar intervertebral disc and trapping of the facet joints are generally believed to be causes of acute low back pain. But it is estimated that the number of patients suffering from low back pain due to the sacroiliac joint dysfunction is not low. First of all, it is

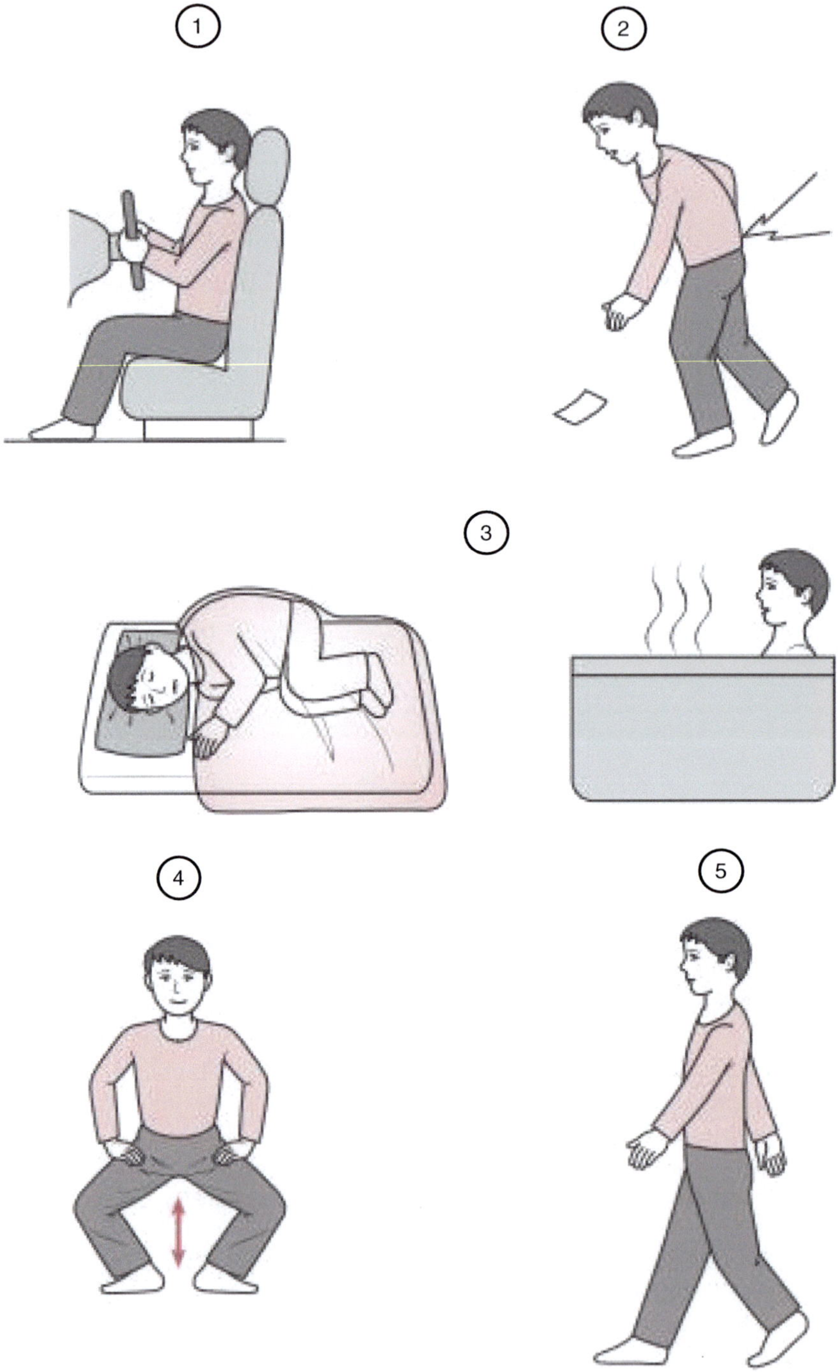

Fig. 7.3 Points to prevent sacroiliac joint disorder. With permission from [8]. ① Avoid working in the same posture for a long time. Take a break during driving or sitting on a chair. ② Be aware of the middle-flexed posture or activity. ③ Do not get tired. Do not let your body cool down. ④ Do squats up and down after taking a bath or in the morning. ⑤ Take an active walk

necessary to recognize that the semi-flexion posture is a dangerous posture. However, in daily life, as avoiding the semi-flexion posture is impossible, it is important to concentrate and be conscious of what you try to do, when it comes to this posture.

The following fact let us understand that remaining conscious is truly effective. It is rare that a weightlifter who lifts more than 100 kg in middle-flexed posture will have low back pain, but there are some housekeepers who develop pain when they simply use a vacuum cleaner while thinking about things such as tonight's dinner. From this fact, it is thought that the human defense mechanism works while only being conscious of lifting a burden. It is important to be attracted when straining not only in the middle-flexed posture but also during any work.

7.3.1.3 Do Not Get Tired, Do Not Let Your Body Cool Down

Because fatigue in the muscles around the low back and the pelvis increases the burden on the SIJs, it is necessary to rest and restore these muscles. Sleeping on your side with the knee bent is effective.

In addition, as patients with SIJ disorder complain of worsening pain when making the SIJ is cooled down, it is often effective to warm the SIJ by taking a bath or using disposable body warmers and Chinese herbal medicines that may improve blood circulation.

7.3.1.4 Do Squats Up and Down After Bathing or in the Morning

It is thought that squats up and down, which the author designed by taking a hint from squats done by the sumo wrestlers, is effective for improving movement of the SIJ. I encourage patients to do this after bathing or in the morning. They will certainly have a feeling of improvement after the exercises.

7.3.1.5 Active Walking

Lack of walking contributes to an increase in sacroiliac joint disorder. It seems that by walking, the muscles supporting the pelvis and lower limbs are strengthened in well-balanced manner. We experienced that the patients who often walked actively did not have recurring SIJ disorder.

7.3.2 Physical Therapy for Stabilizing the SIJ

Effective physical therapy for SIJ disorder has not yet been established.

It is indicated that the transversus abdominis muscle and gluteus maximus muscle are important in stabilizing the SIJ [3, 4].

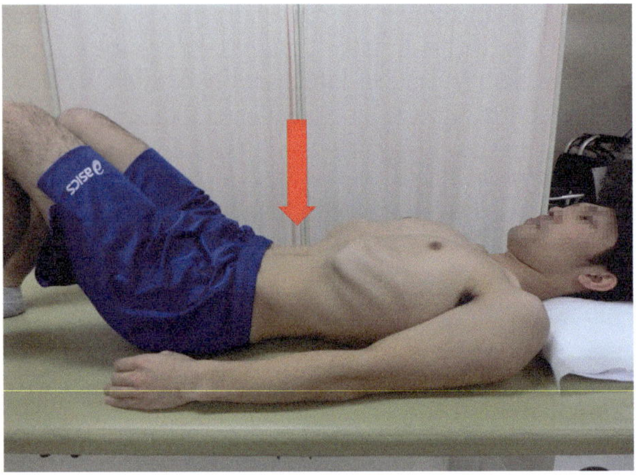

Fig. 7.4 Draw-in exercise for SIJ stabilization. Draw-in of the lower abdominal wall while expiring in the supine position produces the most activity of the transversus abdominis

7.3.2.1 Exercise for the Transversus Abdominis Muscle

Draw-In: Inward Movement of the Lower Abdominal Wall (Fig. 7.4)
Inward movement of the lower abdominal wall in the supine position (draw-in) produces the most independent activity of the transversus abdominis relative to the other abdominal muscles (rectus abdominis and oblique externus abdominis) [5].

Moreover, Takaki et al. [6] indicated that the transversus abdominis showed higher activity than that of the other muscles while performing an active posterior pelvic tilting motion in a standing position. Thus, the draw-in exercise during posterior pelvic tilting motion is thought to be more effective.

7.3.2.2 Exercise for the Gluteus Maximus Muscle

The gluteus maximus muscles lay across and support the SIJ [4]. It has been reported that the onset of the oblique internus abdominis muscle, multifidus muscle, and gluteus maximus muscle was delayed in patients with SIJ disorder during hip flexion while standing [7].

> **Key Message: Bridge Exercise** (Fig. 7.5)
> The draw-in exercise selectively promotes activity of the transversus abdominis. On the other hand, the bridge exercise is performed in order to contract the local muscles (transversus abdominis, multifidus, etc.) and the global muscles (rectus abdominis muscle and oblique externus abdominis muscle or gluteus maximus) together. As for a training position, back bridge exercise, while sustaining a raised limb position, is effective for training the gluteus maximus muscle and the multifidus muscles (Fig. 7.5a). Elbow-toe bridge exercise is effective for training the gluteus maximus muscle and the transversus abdominis muscle (Fig. 7.5b).

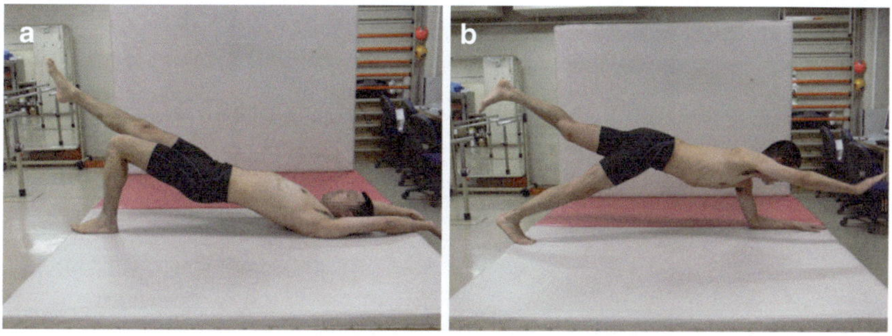

Fig. 7.5 Bridge exercise. With permission from [8]. (**a**) Back bridge exercise (the training of the gluteus maximus muscle and the multifidus muscles). (**b**) Elbow-toe bridge exercise (the training of the transversus abdominis muscle and the gluteus maximus muscle)

7.3.2.3 Preventing Contracture of the Rectus Femoris Muscle or Hamstring Muscle

Contracture of the rectus femoris or hamstring muscle, both of which are attached to the innominate, can apply rotational shearing force on the SIJ. Therefore, flexibility in the muscles and ligaments around the hip joint is important for decreasing rotational shearing force on the SIJ.

7.3.3 Squatting Exercise for Maintaining the Function of the SIJ

I would like to introduce the following exercise that is effective for maintaining the function of the SIJ.

7.3.3.1 Exercises: The Patient Squats While Keeping Your Legs Open

First rotate both feet externally to the maximum while going down and up the back vertically as straight as possible. Perform this exercise several times while holding something with your hands to keep stable (Fig. 7.6a–c). Then, twist your low back and dip one shoulder inward. Perform this exercise alternately between both shoulders 2–3 times (Fig. 7.6d, e). The author advises patients do this exercise after bathing or in the morning. In addition, the posture of sumo wrestler which lowers the low back seems to be effective for maintaining and normalizing joint function.

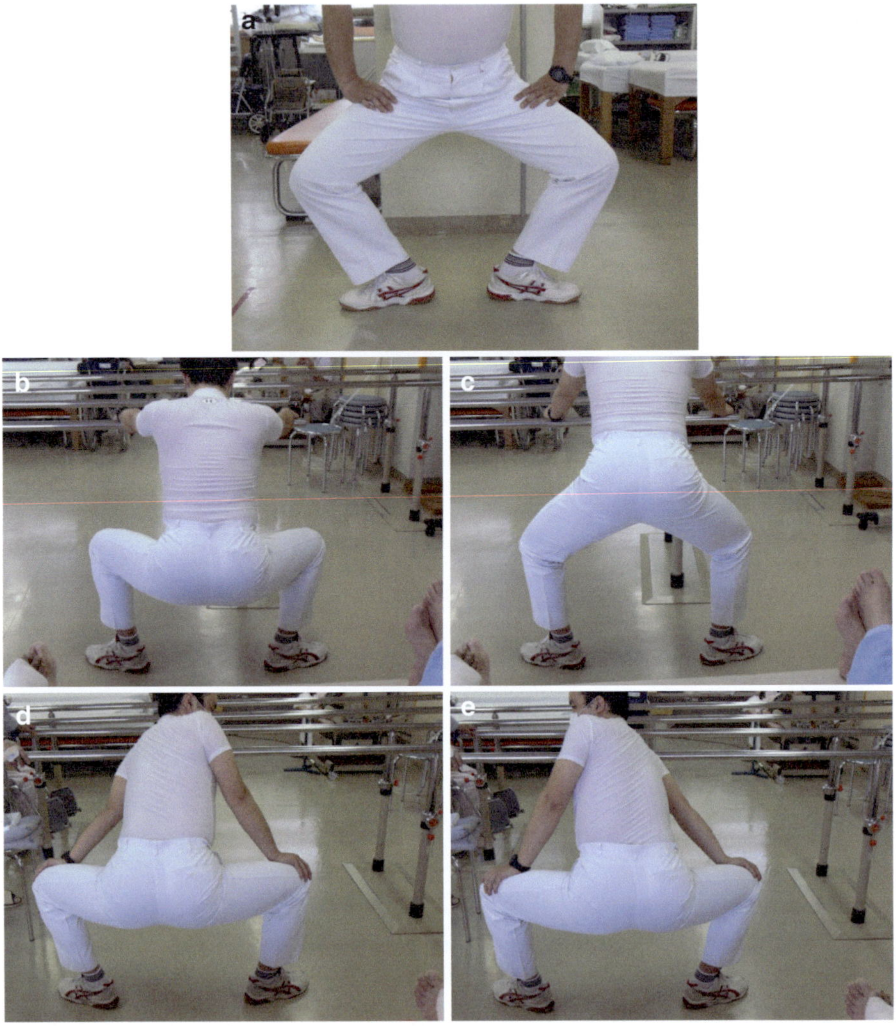

Fig. 7.6 Exercise of squatting up and down with legs open. With permission from [8]. (**a**) Rotate both feet externally to the maximum. (**b**) Hold something with your hands and perform going down and up (**c**) the back vertically as straight as possible several times. (**d**) Twist your low back and dip one shoulder inward. (**e**) Perform this exercise alternately between both shoulders 2–3 times

References

1. Kapandji IA. The trunk and the vertebral column. In: The physiology of the joints, vol. 3. Edinburgh: Churchill Livingstone; 1974.
2. Irion JM. Use of the gym ball in rehabilitation of spinal dysfunction. Orthop Phys Ther Clin North Am. 1992;1:375–98.

3. Richardson CA, et al. The relation between the transversus abdominis muscles, SIJ mechanics, and low back pain. Spine. 2002;27:399–405.
4. Hungerford B, et al. Altered patterns of pelvic bone motion determined in subjects with posterior pelvic pain using skin markers. Clin Biomech. 2004;19:456–64.
5. Urquhart DM, et al. Abdominal muscle recruitment during a range of voluntary exercises. Man Ther. 2005;10:144–53.
6. Takaki S, et al. Analysis of the muscle activity during anterior and posterior pelvic tilting. Gothenburg: The International Society for the Study of the Lumbar Spine; 2010.
7. Hungerford B, et al. Evidence of altered lumbopelvic muscle recruitment in the presence of SIJ pain. Spine. 2003;28:1593–600.
8. Murakami E. Sacroiliac joint pain: undiagnosed low back pain. Tokyo: Nankodo; 2012. (in Japanese).

8 The Tragedy of Low Back Pain that Cannot Be Diagnosed from Images

8.1 Case 1: SIJ Disorder that Was Almost Performed Posterior Lumbar Interbody Fusion (PLIF)

[53-year-old female]

Chief Complaint
Right gluteal pain and numbness of the inside of the lower right leg

Current Medical History
The patient was diagnosed as having pain from lumbar disc herniation by a local doctor (Fig. 8.1a, b). She had received epidural injections for nearly a year. However, her pain did not improve and her daily life became difficult. The doctor recommended the L4–L5 posterior lumbar interbody fusion (PLIF). The surgery was scheduled. However, because she had anxiety about the surgery, she visited JCHO Sendai Hospital to obtain a second opinion.

First Visit Finding
Using one finger, she indicated the region around PSIS as the most painful area. The SIJ shear test and the Gaenslen's test were positive, and tenderness on the PSIS/sacrotuberous ligament was present, which are typical of SIJ disorder (Fig. 8.1c).

Progress
At her first visit, her disease was suspected to be SIJ disorder according to these findings, so SIJ injection under fluoroscopy was performed twice (Fig. 8.1d). As a result, her scores on the visual analogue scale (VAS, 84 → 24) and the Roland-Morris.

Disability Questionnaire (RDQ, 18 → 7) both improved, and she could return to work.

Lessons Learned
Lumbar disc herniation visible on MRI is not always a cause of pain.

E. Murakami, *Sacroiliac Joint Disorder*,
https://doi.org/10.1007/978-981-13-1807-8_8

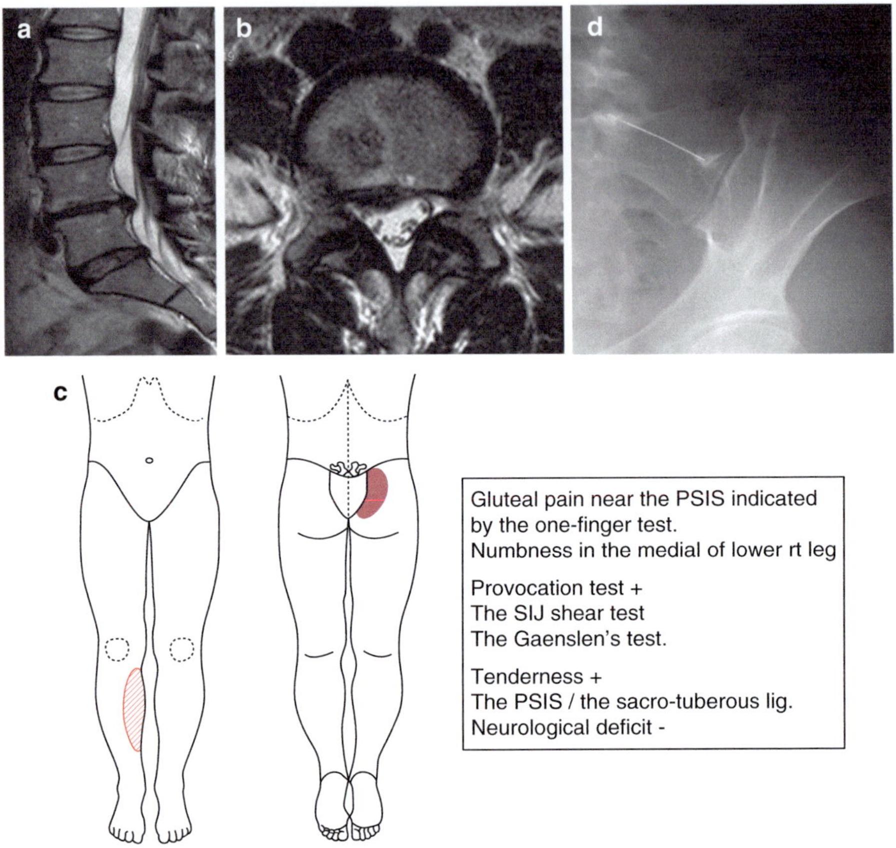

Fig. 8.1 (**a**) Sagittal view of the lumbar spine on MRI shows L4/L5 disc herniation (arrow). (**b**) Coronal view of the lumbar spine on MRI; L4/L5 disc herniation is found on the right side. (**c**) Pain area and physical findings; highlighted area indicates area of numbness. (**d**) View of needle insertion; pain was relieved after receiving an SIJ injection twice. With permission from [1]

Numbness localized to the inside of the lower leg rarely occurs in lumbar nerve root injuries.

It is necessary to thoroughly examine whether findings on the image reveal the pain or not by considering the nerve root block and neurological findings, without being deceived by the image.

8.2 Case 2: SIJ Disorder with a Chief Complaint of Groin Pain

[61-year-old female]

Chief Complaint
Left groin pain and left back gluteal pain

Current Medical History
When she lifted an oil can 1 month prior, left groin pain and left back gluteal pain developed. Though she consulted a gynecologist, a urologist, and a gastroenterologist to find the cause of her abdominal pain, it remained unknown. In order to confirm the presence of orthopedic disease, she was introduced to our department.

First Visit Finding
The one-finger test indicated pain near the PSIS; the SIJ shear test and the Patrick's test were positive. External rotation of the left hip joint was limited. In addition, tenderness on PSIS, the long posterior sacroiliac ligament, and the iliac muscle was present. She could not sit, which is indicative of SIJ disorder (Fig. 8.2a).

Progress
SIJ injection under fluoroscopy was performed three times. Her scores on the pain scale (9 → 2), VAS (74 → 32), and RDQ (16 → 7) all improved.

Lessons Learned
- Groin pain is a characteristic of SIJ disorder even if there is no abnormality in the hip joint on the image.
- Pain from the lower abdomen to the groin region should primarily imply SIJ disorder. Also, many cases cause restriction in the range of motion of the hip joint due to dysfunction of the SIJ.
- It is necessary to recognize that some patients with SIJ disorder are among those who consult physicians or gynecologists due to a chief complaint of abdominal pain.

8.3 Case 3: Hip Osteoarthrosis: Pain Was Relieved After SIJ Injection

[76-year-old female]

Chief Complaint
Left groin pain

Current Medical History
Left hip osteoarthrosis has been indicated. Left groin pain appeared 3 years prior. The patient visited the hospital to make up her mind regarding total hip arthroplasty (THA).

First Visit Findings
The area of the pain was the left groin and the buttocks. On X-ray, the joint cleft had completely disappeared (Fig. 8.3a). However, the sacroiliac joint shear test and Gaenslen's test were positive, and tenderness on the PSIS/iliac muscle was present. Tenderness on the Scarpa triangle was negative. It was a finding typical of SIJ disorder (Fig. 8.3b).

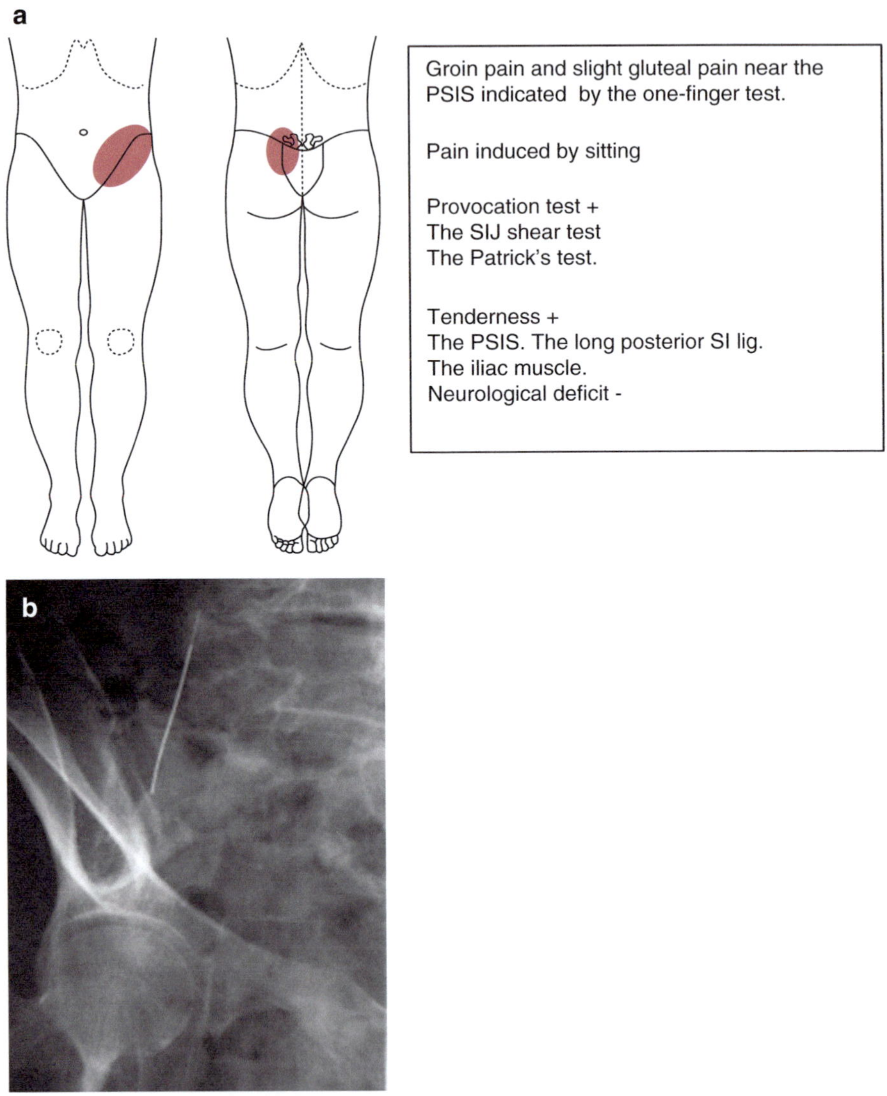

Fig. 8.2 (**a**) Pain area and physical findings. (**b**) X-ray of a needle insertion; after an SIJ injection was performed three times, pain was relieved. With permission from [1]

Progress
SIJ injection resulted in more than 80% pain relief.

Lessons Learned
If there is a finding of hip osteoarthrosis on the X-ray image, we might easily conclude that groin pain is also derived from hip arthrosis. It is not uncommon that groin pain can be relieved after the SIJ injection in such cases. It is necessary to

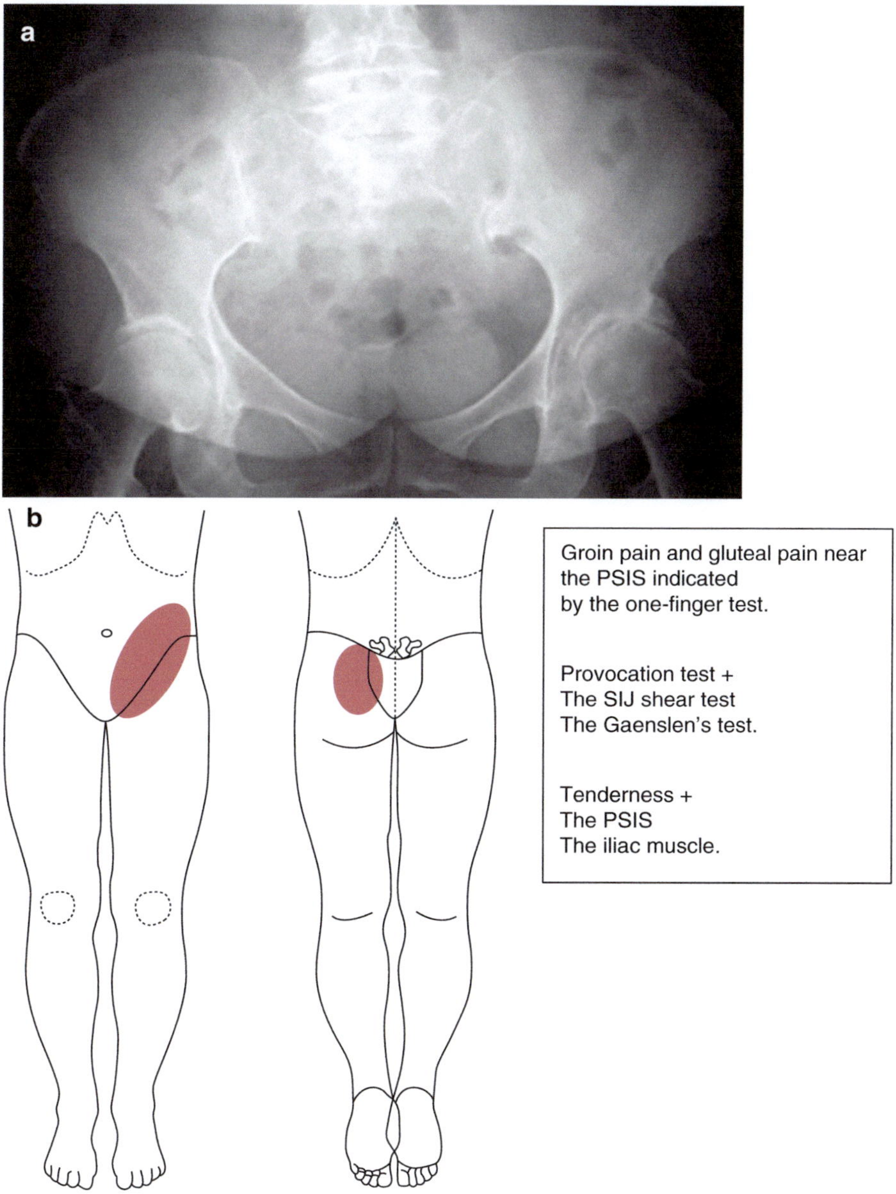

Fig. 8.3 (**a**) AP view of the hip joint on X-ray. (**b**) Pain area and physical findings. With permission from [1]

recognize that groin pain is not only derived from hip osteoarthrosis but also from SIJ disorder.

8.4 Case 4: SIJ Disorder Developed After Total Hip Arthroplasty (THA)

[63-year-old female]

Chief Complaint
Right groin pain and right lower back pain

Current Medical History
THA was performed for right hip osteoarthrosis (Fig. 8.4a). Postoperatively, right groin pain and right lower back pain appeared. As SIJ disorder was suspected, the patient was introduced to our department.

First Visit Findings
The pain area was the right groin and the right back. The sacroiliac joint shear test and Gaenslen's test were positive, and tenderness on the iliac muscle was present, showing findings typical of SIJ disorder (Fig. 8.4b).

Progress
Pain was relieved by several sacroiliac joint injections.

Lessons Learned
- In THA, the joint capsule and ligament of the hip joint are resected, so joint sensory receptors are lacking.
- It is considered rare for a patient to develop hip joint pain after surgery [1].
- When groin pain appears after THA, we should suspect that the pain is firstly originating from the sacroiliac joint, not from around the hip joint.

8.5 Case 5: SIJ Disorder Complicated with Lumbar Disc Herniation

[30-year-old male]

Chief Complaint
Pain from the right buttock to the posterior thigh and the posterior lower leg (Fig. 8.5a)

Current Medical History
Due to right L5/S1 disc herniation, we realized the limitations of injection therapy. We performed surgery for disc herniation. After surgery, pain in the right buttock,

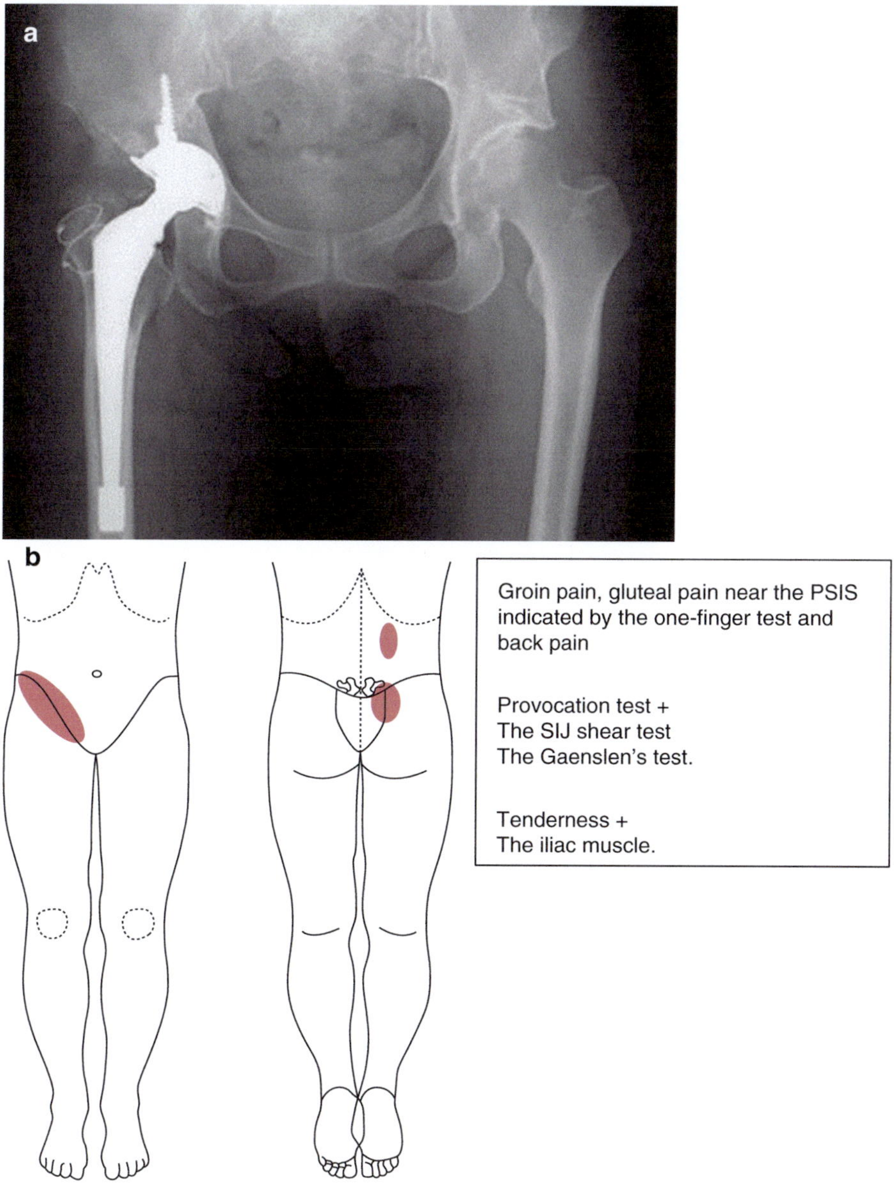

Fig. 8.4 (**a**) AP view of the hip joint on X-ray (after right THA). (**b**) Painful area and physical findings. With permission from [1]

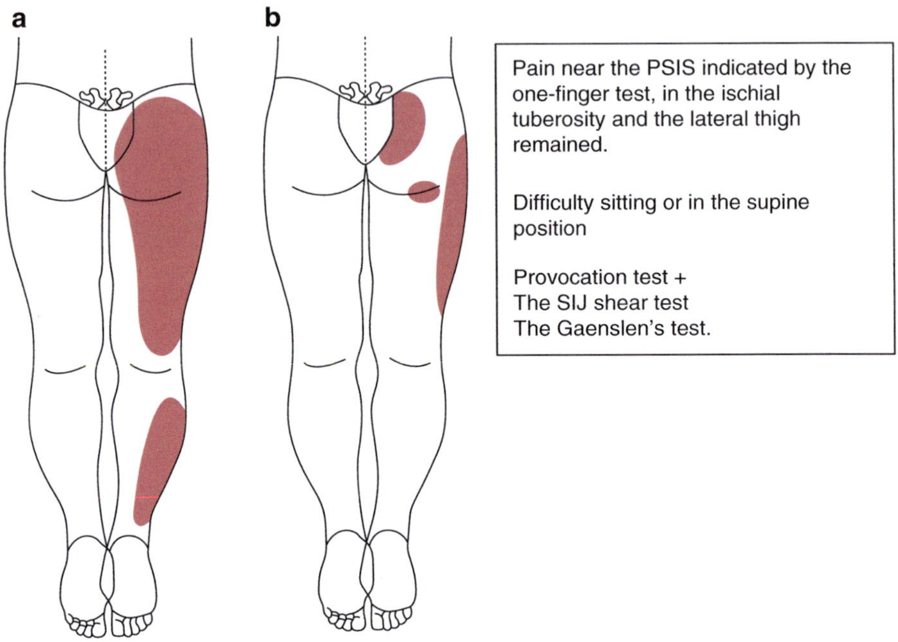

Fig. 8.5 (**a**) Pre-op pain area. (**b**) Pain area and physical findings post-op. With permission from [1]

the ischial tuberosity, and the lateral thigh remained. Initially, we suspected some remnant of the lumbar disc herniation and performed a right nerve root block, but the symptoms were not relieved.

Progress

When we heard a detailed description of the area of pain indicated by the patient, he had pain around the PSIS and the ischial tuberosity (which are characteristic of SIJ disorder), and the patient said that he could not lie in a supine position or sit. Also, the one-finger test indicated the area near PSIS. The sacroiliac joint shear test and Gaenslen's test were also positive, showing findings of SIJ disorder (Fig. 8.5b). A SIJ injection was performed three times, and pain was relieved.

Lessons Learned

- This case is one with the possibility of unnecessary reoperation. The symptoms remaining after surgery were not caused by the nerve root being compressed by lumbar disc herniation but rather by SIJ disorder.
- If we know that pain around the PSIS and ischial tuberosity are characteristic of SIJ disorder, then it is not difficult to find this. Furthermore, if there is an appeal from the patient that the supine position and sitting position are difficult, you should immediately suspect SIJ disorder.

It is important to keep in mind during examination that the number of cases of SIJ disorder associated with lumbar disc herniation and lumbar spinal stenosis are not few.

8.6 Case 6: SIJ Disorder Developed After Surgery for Lumbar Spinal Stenosis

[73-year-old male]

Chief Complaint
Left gluteal and groin pain and left lateral leg pain

Current Medical History
There was a finding of lumbar spinal stenosis in MRI, and because the patient's walking ability was limited to 50 m due to intermittent claudication, L4/L5 partial laminectomy was performed. After surgery, the symptoms improved, but at 3 months after surgery, left gluteal and groin pain and left lateral leg pain appeared, which made it difficult to walk. A left L5 nerve root injury was suspected. Though root block was performed, the pain was not relieved. Because the SIJ injection was partially effective, he was introduced to our department for diagnosis and treatment.

First Visit Findings
The sacroiliac joint shear test was positive, and tenderness on the PSIS and iliac muscle was present. Both sitting position and supine position were difficult, showing findings typical of SIJ disorder (Fig. 8.6).

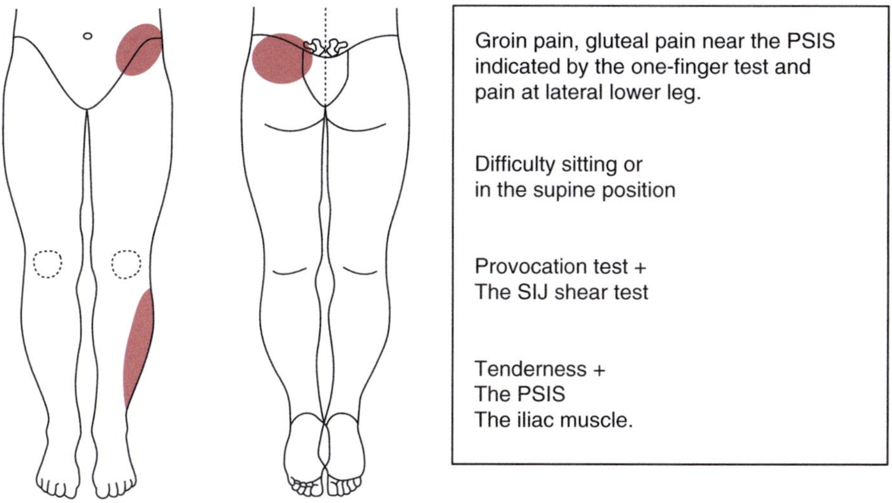

Fig. 8.6 Pre-op pain area. Groin pain, gluteal pain and pain at lateral lower leg were indicated. With permission from [1]

Progress
SIJ injection reduced left gluteal and groin pain, but left lateral leg pain remained. The lateral leg pain was reproduced on the left L5 nerve root block, so a reoperation was performed. A strong adhesion of L5 nerve root was noted during surgery, and the pain was relieved after exfoliation of the adhesion.

Lessons Learned
- A combination of SIJ disorder and nerve root adhesion developed after surgery. Left buttock and groin pain were originated from the SIJ; on the other hand, left lateral leg pain was due to nerve root adhesion. It is not unusual that a combination of SIJ disorder and nerve root adhesion develops after lumbar surgery.
- When there is pain that cannot be explained from nerve root injury, it is important to conduct a medical examination while keeping the possibility of SIJ disorder in mind.

8.7 Case 7: SIJ Disorder in Which Symptoms Disappeared After Removal of Lumbar Disc Herniation

[30-year-old male]

Chief Complaint
Right buttock and posterior leg pain

Current Medical History
- After removal of the right L5/S1 disc herniation for right low back and leg pain was performed, the initial pain disappeared. But after lifting a heavy thing, new pain developed in the right buttock and posterior leg pain.
- MRI scans showed right re-herniated disc at L5/S1 (Fig. 8.7a). We firstly suspected a nerve root injury, but S1 nerve root block was not so effective. So, the patient was introduced to our department for the purpose of detailed examination.

First Visit Findings
The sacroiliac joint shear test was positive, and tenderness on PSIS, iliac muscle, and sacrotuberous ligament was present. SIJ disorder was suspected (Fig. 8.7b).

Progress
After SIJ injection, the right buttock pain was temporarily relieved, but the right posterior leg pain remained. Because the pain had disappeared following the S1 nerve root block for a few hours, we surgically removed the L5/S1 disc herniation. After the surgery, not only the posterior leg pain but also the buttock pain was

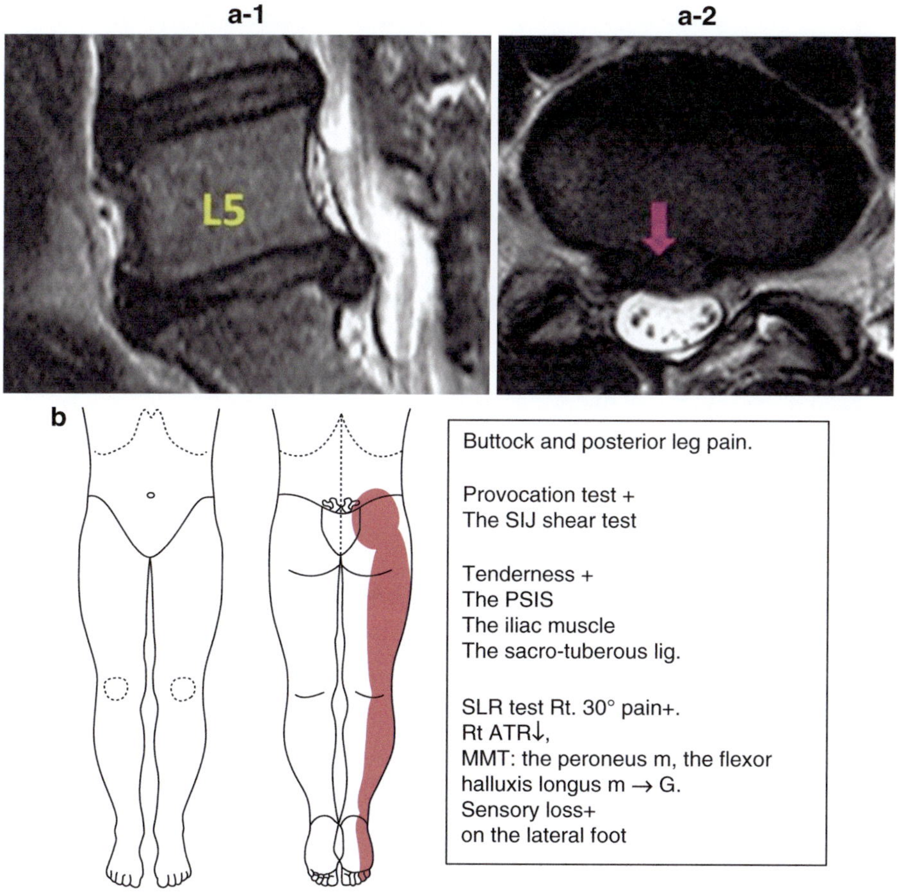

Fig. 8.7 (**a**) MRI of lumbar spine; L5/S1 disc herniation (arrow) is found (**a-1**, sagittal view; **a-2**, coronal view). (**b**) Pre-op pain area. With permission from [1]

relieved. Moreover, the SIJ shear test came up negative, and tenderness on the PSIS, iliac muscle, and sacrotuberous ligament also disappeared.

Lessons Learned

- After removal of L5/S1 disc herniation, not only the posterior leg pain but also symptoms of sacroiliac joint disorder diminished. It is a fact that there was SIJ disorder before surgery, because the tenderness points on such locations as the PSIS and iliac muscle, as well as the buttock pain, were relieved following SIJ injection.
- Taking this phenomenon into consideration, it seems that a load on the SIJ may be reduced after herniectomy.
- [See Column "The Theory that the Sacroiliac Joint Functions Like a Dam."]

8.8 Case 8: SIJ Disorder Developed After Lumbar Spinal Fusion

[72-year-old female]

Chief Complaint
Pain around both PSIS and bilateral groin and anterior thigh pain

Current Medical History
- L4–L5 PLIF was performed (Fig. 8.8a, b). After the surgery, lower leg pain was relieved, but gradually pain around both PSIS and bilateral groin and anterior thigh pain developed.
- In addition to the front of the thigh, she experienced isolated pain in the knee and the inside of the right lower thigh. Also, on both sides of the SIJ, the sacroiliac joint shear test was positive, and tenderness on both iliac muscles and right sacrotuberous ligament was present. SIJ disorder was suspected (Fig. 8.8c).

Progress
SIJ injection relieved pain for 1–2 weeks, so we continued treatment at the outpatient clinic.

Lessons Learned
- The occurrence of neighboring intervertebral disorders after lumbar spinal fusion is well known. It is considered that the disorders will be caused by an increase of the load into neighboring vertebral bodies following the fusion.
- Unoki et al. [1] reported that the incidence of SIJ disorder after lumbar spinal fusion was found in 8.4% of cases of fixed fusion including the sacral bone or long fusion. The incidence was more than in those without fusion of the sacral bone or with short fusion.
- It is important to examine patients while recognizing that there are not a few SIJ disorders, including buttock pain, which develop after lumbar spinal fusion.

8.9 Case 9: SIJ Disorder: Pain Was Relieved After Removing the Instruments Used for Lumbar Spinal Fusion

[37-year-old female]

Chief Complaint
Left gluteal pain

Current Medical History
She received L4–L5 PLIF for lumbar disc herniation. After surgery, her back pain gradually increased, and then she received L4–S1PLIF (Fig. 8.9a, b). Left buttock pain gradually developed. Because SIJ injection was effective for the patient's left

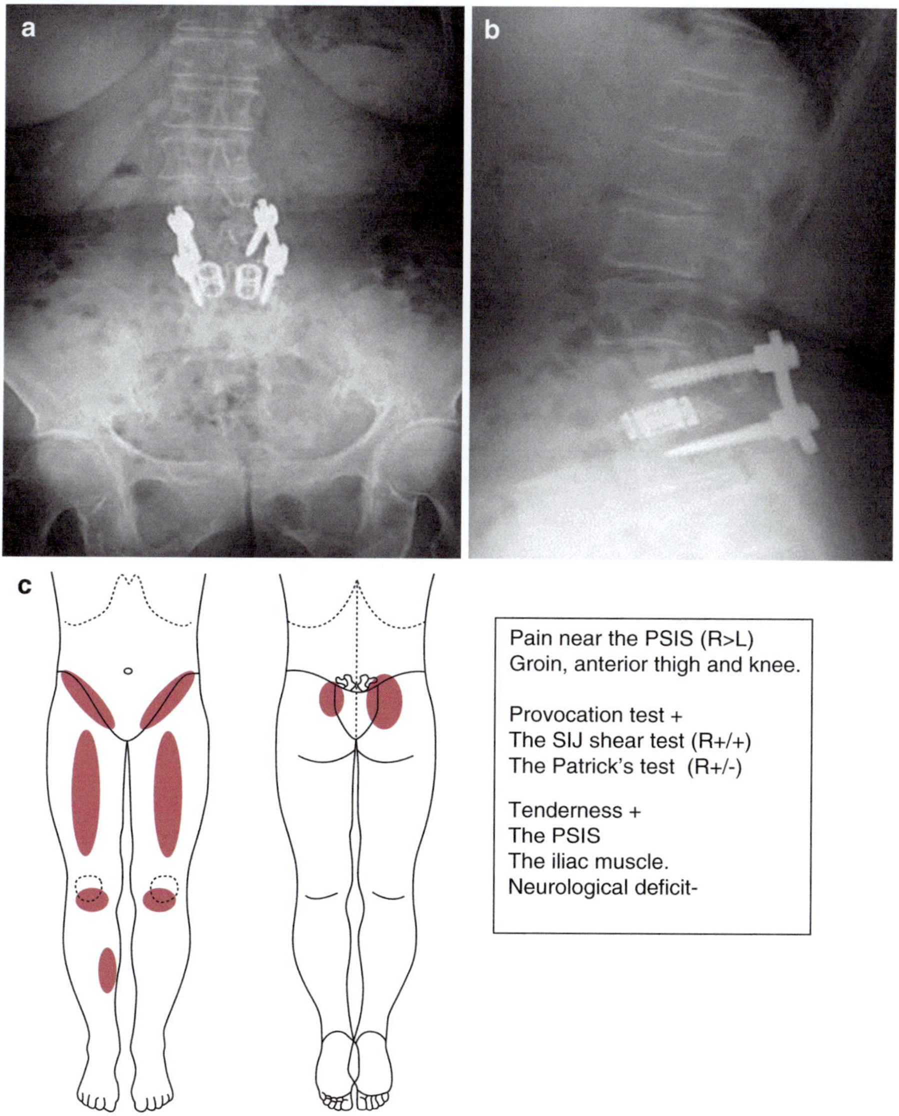

Fig. 8.8 (**a**) AP view of lumbar spine on X-ray. (**b**) Lateral view of lumbar spine. (**c**) Painful area and physical findings. With permission from [1]

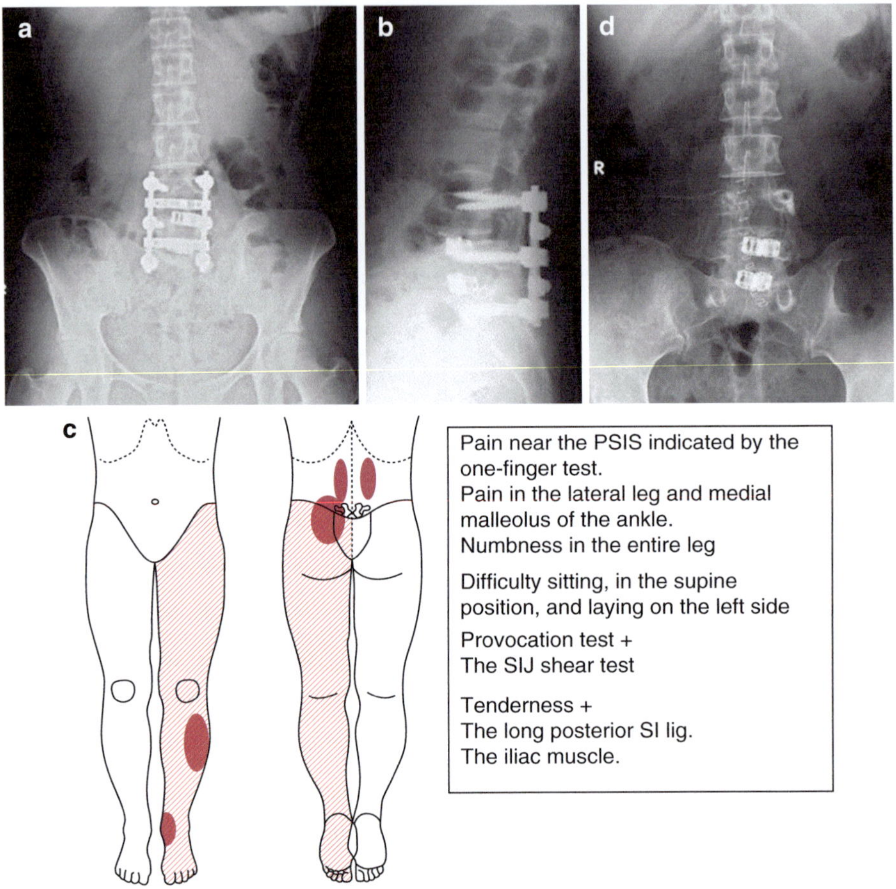

Fig. 8.9 (**a**) AP view of lumbar spines on X-ray. (**b**) Lateral view of lumbar spines on X-ray. (**c**) Pain area and physical findings; highlighted area indicates area of numbness. (**d**) AP view of lumbar spines on X-ray (after removing internal instruments). With permission from [1]

buttock pain, the injections were performed more than 50 times. However, the effects of the injections were temporary, so she was introduced to our department.

First Visit Findings

There was pain around the left PSIS and the left lateral leg and medial malleolus of the ankle. Dull numbness was seen throughout the left leg. Lying supine, lying on the left side, and sitting were difficult. The one-finger test also indicated the area near the PSIS; the sacroiliac joint shear test was positive, and tenderness on the long posterior SI ligament and iliac muscle was present, which were typical findings of SI disorder (Fig. 8.9c).

Progress

- Conservative therapies (SIJ injection, AKA-Hakata method) were tried for more than 3 months, but symptoms did not improve. Therefore, suspecting that rigid lumbar fusion including the sacral bones was causing SIJ disorder, we removed the instruments for lumbar internal fusion (Fig. 8.9d). After the removal, SIJ pain diminished.
- Her score on the pain scale improved from 10 to 4; numbness also decreased.

Lessons Learned

- In theory, mobility of the lumbar spine does not change, even if internal fixation is removed, because bone grafting and fixation should be complete. However, pain is actually relieved after the removal of internal fixation. There is a possibility that the rigid fixation of the lumbar spine by metals suppresses minor movement of a living body, which can be recovered after removing them. And so, the mechanical stress on the SIJ is dispersed somewhat. Accordingly, SIJ pain is diminished.
- Because an increase of SIJ disorder after posterior lumbar spinal fusion is expected, it is necessary that surgical indications for lumbar spinal fusion by metals should be more strict.

8.10 Case 10: SIJ Disorder: Occurring After Thoracolumbar-Compressed Fracture

[80-year-old female]

Chief Complaint

Back pain and left gluteal pain

Current Medical History

One month ago after a fall from a chair, back pain and pain in the left gluteal area gradually appeared. The pain increased strongly with movement; walking was difficult.

Initial Visit Findings

- Multiple compressed fractures were observed mainly in the thoracolumbar transition area (Th 11, Th 12) on MRI (Fig. 8.10a). Although there was tenderness in the spinous process near the compression fracture, left gluteal pain was far from the site of the compression fracture. Furthermore pain was indicated at the PSIS by the one-finger test, and the sacroiliac joint shear test was positive.
- So we suspected a merger with SIJ disorder (Fig. 8.10b).

Progress

Two SIJ injections relieved the pain. Rising from a chair and walking were now possible.

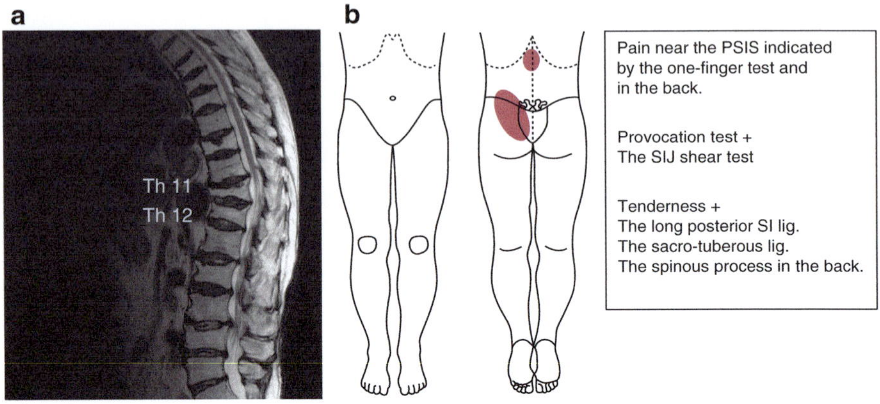

Fig. 8.10 (**a**) Sagittal view of thoracic spine on MRI. (**b**) Pain area and physical findings

Lessons Learned

- Mergers of SIJ disorder after compressed fractures of the thoracolumbar area are not rare. It is considered that the gravity line shifts more forward, and the burden on the SIJ increases following the progress of thoracic kyphosis.
- It is important to examine a patient not only with the intent to take care of the site of the compressed fracture but with a recognition that SIJ disorder may emerge after compressed fractures of the thoracolumbar area.

8.11 Case 11: SIJ Disorder: Weakness of Lower Limb, Which Developed Due to SIJ Disorder, Made Walking Difficult

[19-year-old male]

Chief Complaint
Weakness of the left lower limb

Current Medical History
After twisting his low back 1 month ago, weakness of the left thigh gradually emerged. He could not bear weight or walk. The case was introduced to our department.

First Visit Findings
On the MRI, the lumbar vertebrae were normal (Fig. 8.11a). Lumbo-gluteal pain was mild. Although weakness was seen in the iliopsoas muscle and the quadriceps muscle, there was no obvious neurological deficit. Also, the sacroiliac joint shear test was negative, but tenderness on the iliac muscle, long posterior sacroiliac ligament, and sacrotuberous ligament was present (Figs. 8.8, 8.9, 8.10, and 8.11b).

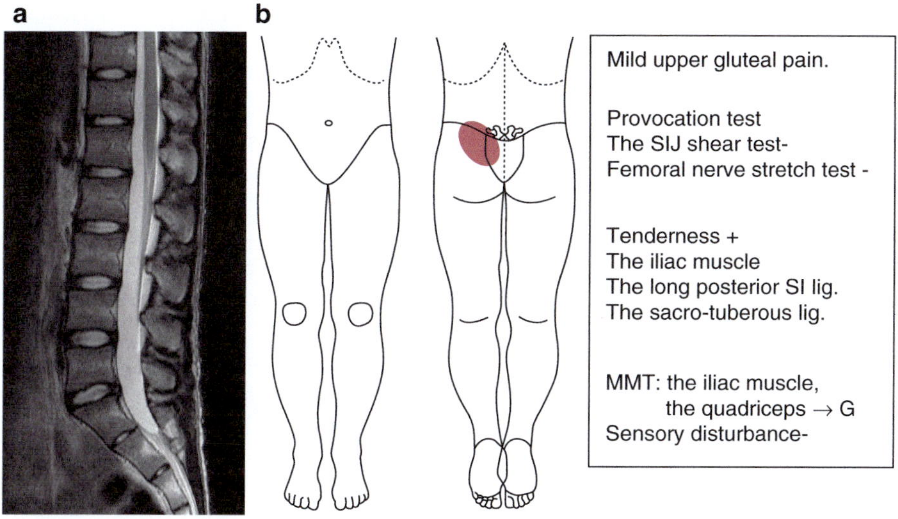

Fig. 8.11 (**a**) Sagittal view of lumbar spine on MRI. (**b**) Pain area and physical findings. With permission from [1]

Progress

SIJ injection was performed, suspecting the weakness was due to SIJ disorder. After the injection, he could immediately take a step forward and was able to walk after three injections.

Lessons Learned

- Initially, I suspected femoral nerve palsy, but the weakness of the thigh was due to SIJ disorder.
- There are patients with SIJ disorder that fall since their feet do not actually go forward, despite their intention of taking a step forward.
- As a mechanism of this weakness, it is conceivable that the tone of soft tissue and muscles decreases due to the lack of joint reflex, so at the moment when the patients intend to step forward, it does not work (see Table 2.2).

8.12 Case 12: SIJ Disorder Diagnosed as Psychogenic Pain

[24-year-old female]

Chief Complaint

Left buttock and left groin pain

Current Medical History

Left buttock and left groin pain gradually appeared 4 years prior. Her disease was diagnosed as lumbar disc disorder at several other hospitals. However, MRI findings in the lumbar region were unclear, and epidural blocks were not effective. When she visited a psychiatrist under suspicion of psychogenic pain, her intellectual ability was determined to be low (IQ 80) and to have a biased personality structure, and she was diagnosed with a somato-expressive disorder. However, she was suspected to have SIJ disorder because the pain was temporarily relieved by SIJ injection, and she was introduced to our department.

First Visit Findings

The patient exhibited severe pain in the left buttock and left groin and tightening pain over the whole left lower limb. Therefore, she could not lay in the supine position, sit, or walk. Only the lateral decubitus position on the affected side was comfortable. The one-finger test indicated the PSIS and the sacroiliac joint shear test was positive. Tenderness on the PSIS, long sacroiliac ligament, sacrotuberous ligament, and iliac muscle was also present. Those findings were typical of SIJ disorder (Fig. 8.12a).

Progress

- Though conservative therapies such as SIJ injection and the AKA-Hakata method had been conducted for 16 months, the pain did not improve so much, and her daily activities were restricted. As we realized the limitation of these conservative therapies, a left SIJ anterior fusion and an additional posterior fusion were performed (Fig. 8.12b).
- After surgery, the pain was relieved from 10 to 4 on the pain scale, and she came to be able to sit for no less than 2 h. Within 2 years after surgery, the joint fusion was completed on CT, and she returned to work by walking with a cane (Fig. 8.12c).

Lessons Learned

- The patient was a smart woman who worked as a banker. We learned that there was a possibility that long, severe chronic pain and disability resulted in such a woman being misdiagnosed as having "low intellectual capability" and with a "somato-expressive disorder."
- We believe that the way to avoid such tragedy is to securely diagnose this disease as early as possible.

8.13 Case 13: SIJ Disorder in a Patient Who Was Suspected of Faking His Disease

[30-year-old male]

Chief Complaint

Right groin and buttock pain

Current Medical History

- Two years prior, right groin and right buttock pain appeared without particular reason. In spite of visiting gastroenterology, urology, and orthopedic surgery, no abnormal findings were indicated by those departments. Finally, being suspected

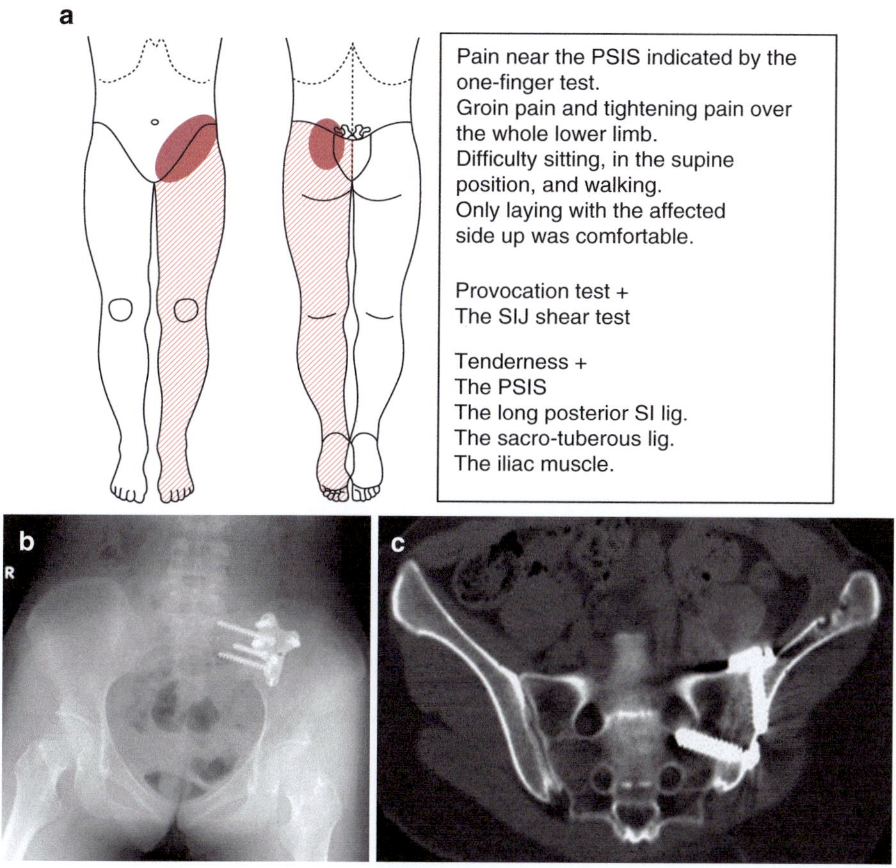

Fig. 8.12 (**a**) Pain area and physical findings. (**b**) AP view of lumbar spines on X-ray (post-op); anterior +posterior fusion. (**c**) Post-op CT findings: joint fusion is confirmed. With permission from [1]

of psychogenic pain, he consulted psychiatry. As a result, he was diagnosed as having a "depressed condition." People in his company and even his family gradually doubted whether he actually suffered from a disease at all.

- Little by little, he began to think about suicide. Since his groin pain was severe, he was introduced to our hospital from a nearby doctor to judge the presence or absence of orthopedic diseases.

First Visit Findings

- The patient exhibited severe pain in the right buttock and groin and accompanying numbness at the lateral leg and the plantar of the foot. Therefore, the supine position, the sitting position, and walking position were difficult. The prone position with a pillow under his chest was the only possible rest position. SIJ shear test and Patrick's test were positive, and tenderness on the PSIS, long sacroiliac ligament, and iliac muscle was also present.
- These were typical of SIJ disorder (Fig. 8.13a).

Progress

There was no sufficient improvement in conservative therapies for more than 6 months, and his daily life was difficult. Because he hoped strongly for surgical therapy, we performed the anterior SIJ fusion (Fig. 8.13b). After surgery, he

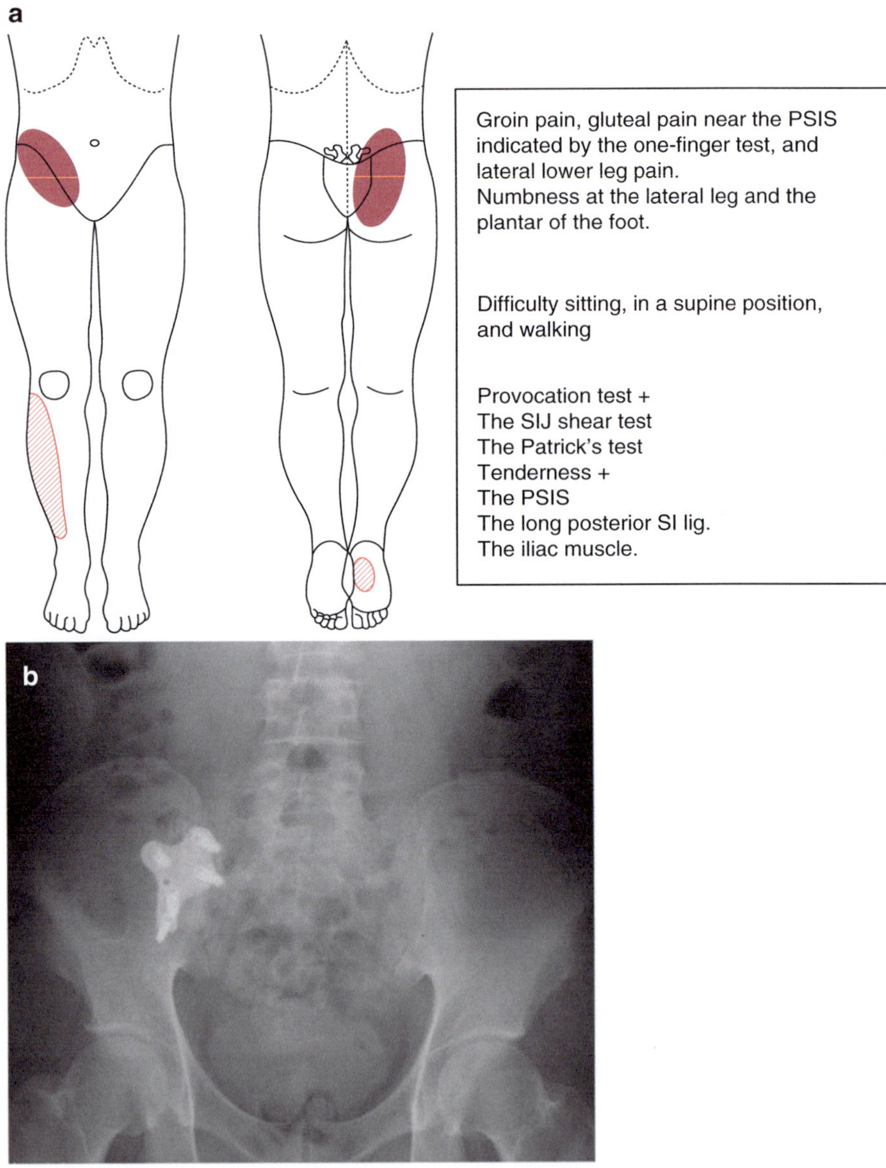

Fig. 8.13 (**a**) Pain area and physical findings; highlighted area indicates area of numbness. (**b**) AP view of the pelvis on X-ray (post-op). With permission from [1]

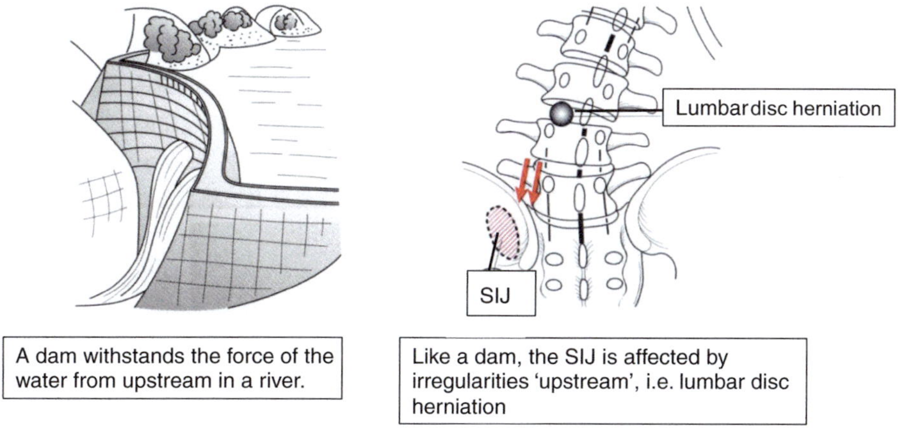

Fig. 8.14 A theory that the sacroiliac joint functions like a dam. With permission from [1]

recognized for the first time in 2 years that he could sleep while looking the ceiling without pain in the supine position. Sitting time and walking time dramatically increased, and he could travel as early as 1 year after surgery. Five years later, he was working as an officer for building and maintenance.

Lessons Learned

Even his family and company’s boss did not understand that he actually had a disease until seeing his pain relief after SIJ fusion. It is supposed that there are many patients with SIJ disorder around the world who go undiagnosed and are mentally driven into a corner by the misunderstanding of people around them.

Key Message: The Theory that the Sacroiliac Joint Functions Like a Dam

As a dam controls the buildup of water upstream in the river, there is a possibility that the SIJ adjusts to the burden caused by disorders such as lumbar disc herniation or lumbar spinal canal stenosis, cranial to the SIJ. As a result, the joint is distorted and develops symptoms.

On the other hand, there is a possibility that the load on the SIJ sometimes decreases, and the disorder of the joint may improve when lumbar disorders are solved by surgery.

However, even if lumbar disorders are cured, the combined SIJ disorder often remains and requires treatment on its own (Fig. 8.14).

Reference

1. Murakami E. Sacroiliac joint pain: undiagnosed low back pain. Tokyo: Nankodo; 2012. (in Japanese).

9 Overview of Our Activities

Abstract

- An annual SIJ seminar for physicians to learn about SIJ disorder has already been held more than 15 times since 2002.
- The Low Back Pain/Sacroiliac Joint Center was opened in the JCHO Sendai Hospital in April 2010.
- The Japanese Sacroiliac Joint Research Society was founded in 2009 with the aim of disseminating the diagnosis and treatment of SIJ disorder. The 8th annual meeting was held in 2017.

9.1 Sacroiliac Joint Seminar

For the purpose of mastering the diagnosis and treatment of sacroiliac joint disorder, we have held an annual SIJ seminar. The 15th seminar was held in 2018. More than 150 doctors, including orthopedic surgeons, neurosurgeons, and pain clinicians, have attended the seminar (Fig. 9.1). They are the core of the Japanese Sacroiliac Joint Research Society. The seminar is made up of various components, such as a lecture, examination of patients, practical training of SIJ injections, and observation of the SIJ fusion. The most popular part of the seminar is the free talking with patients, who have undergone the SIJ fusion, and participating physicians. Listening to patients talk about their experience leading up to the surgery and postoperative changes has a considerable persuasive power in convincing participants that there are patients who suffer from SIJ disorder. This seminar has given its participants a good understanding of the diagnosis and treatment of SIJ disorder.

E. Murakami, *Sacroiliac Joint Disorder*,
https://doi.org/10.1007/978-981-13-1807-8_9

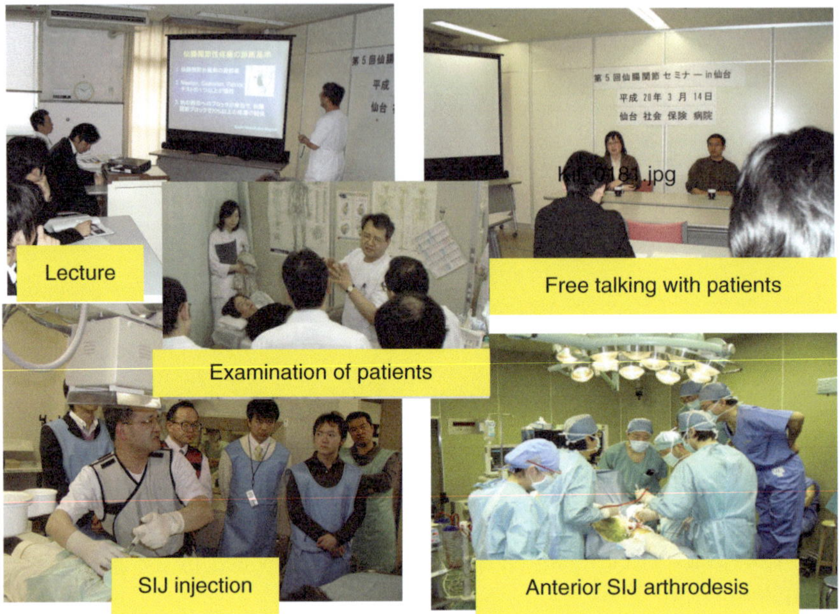

Fig. 9.1 Sacroiliac Joint Seminar

9.2 Low Back Pain and Sacroiliac Joint Center (Fig. 9.2)

As patients were being introduced to us from hospitals all over the country, we decided to open the Low Back Pain/Sacroiliac Joint Center in the JCHO Sendai Hospital in April 2010. It was established with the concept of being the first center nationwide able to totally treat patients with SIJ disorder, using SIJ injections, manual therapy such as the AKA-Hakata method, and arthrodesis as a final remedy. Fifteen years had passed from the time we started treating patients with SIJ disorder to the establishment of the center.

9.3 Japanese Sacroiliac Joint Research Society (Fig. 9.3)

In 2009, the Japanese Sacroiliac Joint Research Association was founded with the aim of disseminating the diagnosis and treatment of pain from the sacroiliac joint. We held the 8th annual meeting in 2017, at which there were 165 participants.

The secretariat is located inside the JCHO Sendai Hospital, and the homepage (http://sentyo-kansetsu.com/) has also been set up. Of course, the annual meeting includes free conversation between patients with SIJ disorder and participants, which is the most popular part of the SIJ seminar, with the message that the annual meeting welcomes not only patients and physicians but anyone interested in joining.

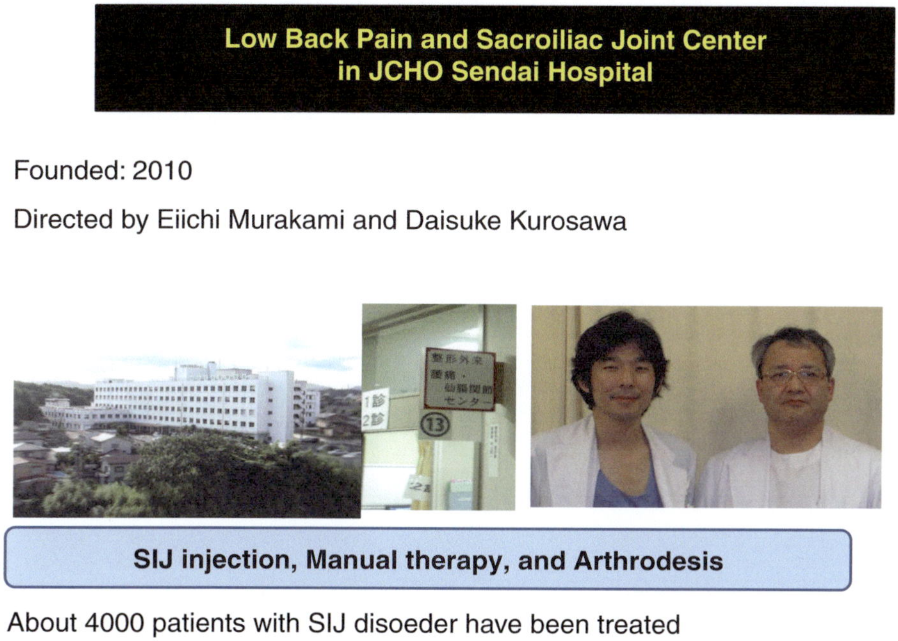

Fig. 9.2 Low Back Pain and Sacroiliac Joint Center in JCHO Sendai Hospital

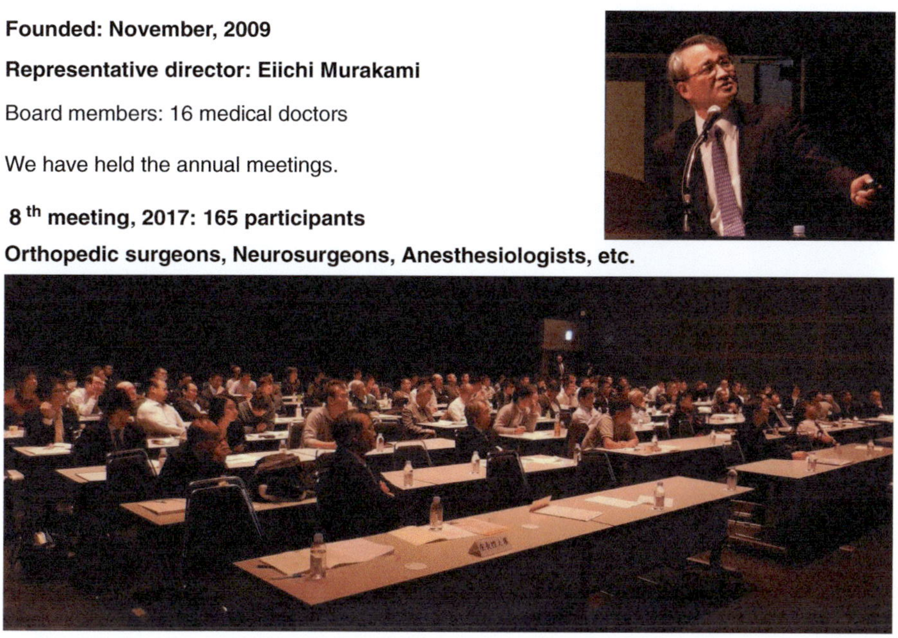
Founded: November, 2009
Representative director: Eiichi Murakami
Board members: 16 medical doctors
We have held the annual meetings.
8 th meeting, 2017: 165 participants
Orthopedic surgeons, Neurosurgeons, Anesthesiologists, etc.

Fig. 9.3 Japanese Sacroiliac Joint Research Society

Glossary

Twenty three years have passed since I met my first patient with SIJ disorder. Since then, not only orthopedic surgeons but also pain clinicians and neurosurgeons have been performing SIJ injections all over Japan.

Some often say "Sacroiliac joint pain is difficult to diagnose because it is hard to capture useful image findings of diseases." This may be especially true of physicians who are accustomed to diagnosing diseases from image findings, but even in the past when imaging equipment was not yet developed, physicians have been able to accurately diagnose many diseases from the patient's physical findings. Moreover, there are many diseases which cannot be detected by image findings, and it is uncertain whether image findings have a direct link to the diagnosis. Thus, it is more important for physicians to not rely too heavily on image findings. If you pay attention to the points of diagnosis mentioned above, I think that it is not difficult to suspect SIJ disorder.

It would bring me happiness if this book is able to provide some suggestions to doctors and patients who are suffering from undiagnosed SIJ disorder. I expect that SIJ disorder will be recognized as a common cause of low back pain and that SIJ injections will become commonplace in treating low back pain.

From now on, while keeping the entomologist Fabre's saying in mind, "Even though various theories give way, the fact that is firmly observed is not broken." I move forward and continue to research SIJ disorder by listening to my patients and paying attention to their physical findings.

E. Murakami, *Sacroiliac Joint Disorder*,
https://doi.org/10.1007/978-981-13-1807-8

Index

E. Murakami, *Sacroiliac Joint Disorder*,
https://doi.org/10.1007/978-981-13-1807-8

MIX
Papier aus verantwortungsvollen Quellen
Paper from responsible sources
FSC® C105338

If you have any concerns about our products,
you can contact us on
ProductSafety@springernature.com

In case Publisher is established outside the EU,
the EU authorized representative is:
Springer Nature Customer Service Center GmbH
Europaplatz 3, 69115 Heidelberg, Germany

Printed by Libri Plureos GmbH
in Hamburg, Germany